THE
TREMOLO
DIARIES

THE TREMOLO DIARIES

LIFE ON THE ROAD AND OTHER DISEASES

JUSTIN CURRIE

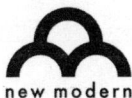

new modern

new modern

First published in the UK in 2025 by New Modern
An imprint of Putman Publishing
Mermaid House, Puddle Dock, Blackfriars, London, EC4V 3DB

@newmodernbooks
@newmodernbooks

Hardback ISBN: 978-1-917923-00-2
eBook ISBN: 978-1-917923-02-6
Audio ISBN: 978-1-917923-01-9

A CIP catalogue record for this book is available in the British Library.

Publishing and editorial: Pete Selby and James Lilford
Typesetting: Marie Doherty

1 3 5 7 9 10 8 6 4 2

New Modern is an imprint of Putman Publishing
www.newmodernbooks.co.uk
www.putmanpublishing.co.uk

MIX
Paper | Supporting
responsible forestry
FSC
www.fsc.org   FSC® C018072

Printed and bound in Great Britain by Clays Ltd, Elcograf S.p.A.

For Emma.
Shall we just start again?

'I'm no good. I'm all worn out. I have been passed from hand to hand. I've had to submit to things that nice young American boys couldn't conceive of in their wildest nightmares. I've lived among the ruins. Armies have marched over me. Armies. I've been debased.'

RITA HAYWORTH AS IRENA IN *FIRE DOWN BELOW*

CAST OF CHARACTERS

AL MARKS – ex-A&M staffer and friend since 1989

ANDY – keyboards since 1988

ANDY P – manager since 2019

BRIAN – guitar tech, with the band since 1988

BUDDY – guitar tech, with the band since 1987

CARLOS – US merch dude

CJ – US bus driver

DOUG – US merch lad

DEREK (MR FUDGE) – tour manager on 2014 US solo tour, and since 2021 with the Dels

FRANÇOIS – monitor man on Barenaked Ladies tour

GA – The Ghastly Affliction

GAVIN – my unreliable right hand

GAV – guitar tech since 2024

HUGH – occasional guitar tech

IAIN – guitarist and songwriter since 1982

JIM – drummer on solo albums and tours since 2007, with Dels since 2021

KRIS – guitarist and songwriter since 1997

LOUIS – Iain's son and occasional tour bus fellow traveller

LUKE – My Love's son

MY LOVE – since 1986, permanently since 2001

SIMON – European tour bus driver since 2022

INTRO

18 January 2022

Ten minutes after seeing the neurologist, I can't get out of the car park. At Glasgow Queen Elizabeth University Hospital, I drive round and around a little multi-storey block for half an hour, unable to discern an exit.

The neurologist, a frank young man whose kind manner was compromised by his surgical mask, had just asked me an odd question.

'Why are you here?'

It had occurred to me then that he was terrified of dropping the P-bomb.

'Well, my GP and I strongly suspect Parkinson's,' I reply.

I can see the man's face, or the sliver of his face that remains uncovered, visibly relax.

'I can do a brain scan today,' he says, 'but we won't find anything. However, in that event, I will not tell you that you *don't* have Parkinson's. Or I can see you in a year.'

I opt for the year of half-knowing, half-hoping.

As I leave his tidy little room, I say, 'So, you're saying I have Parkinson's, but you can't confirm the diagnosis for a year. How do you know?'

'Relax your arms by your side,' he says, and my right hand gently trembles at my hip, as if it's remembering something tricky.

'Now lift your hands to shoulder height.'

The tremor stops.

'That's how.'

So, I begin the year of dread and hope, trapped in a comical maze, in a comical car with a quizzical look on my face. And twelve months later, I sail out of the same place secure in the knowledge I'm ill, and emboldened by the pleasant surprise that they have pills for this sort of thing.

I decide I'm going to keep working, keep touring, keep playing, despite the uneasy feeling that another man is growing inside me, slowly seizing the means of control. It's as if your own shadow has leapt from the ground and buried itself within you. And this shadow has malevolent intent. He may share my shape, but now we're combined, it's a fight to find out who has the most valid claim.

PART ONE

DAY 0, Glasgow Airport
1 June 2023

I'm sitting in Glasgow Airport, contemplating the treacherous wreck of my recent life. The usual snarl of travellers swim around me, unembarrassed by this concerted effort to continue the ruination of Earth's atmosphere with alacrity. Business or pleasure, it's all the same. We don't care and we don't care that we don't care. It's the ghastly affliction.

My own ghastly affliction is evinced by a stiff shoulder and trembling right hand, classic symptoms that something odd is afoot. In my burgeoning infirmity, I'm bound for what will probably be my last major tour with my group Del Amitri, third on the bill on an arduous trek through the circus sheds of America. It feels like our one hundredth trip to the US, the hundredth visit to us, the continent where all this music was born and raised, the font of what is loosely called 'rock'. Us, us, us. Rock's claim to a universal language of collective catharsis and global inclusivity is as bogus as a Tory slogan or religious platitude. We are in nothing together, as the Ghastly Affliction has taught me. We're solo voyagers looking for love and validation. We're as sick as the sea.

The shake in my hand I call Gavin. A traitor who comes and goes and betrays any surge of adrenaline, any passing thought; like a spectre who suddenly appears as a mocking fool, parodying emotions, putting one's secret desires on public display. Gavin is an underminer and an intermittent reminder that I'm ill and unsteady. As lead singer and songwriting leader, steadiness has been my strongest suit. I might be a mediocrity, but I'm always there, reliable and consistent. Now I'm somewhere else, distracted and flaky. The foundations of who I am are weak and watery, like a bad cup of tea. But I can walk around and witness and I can still sing and sway and so, like all musicians, I'm driven by *another* ghastly affliction to play. Because to play is not to work and though we call playing work, it is nothing of the sort. It is the vaunting desire to show feelings and write them in the air, like Beatles and Dylans before us described worlds unseen and emotions not yet experienced. It is the last-ditch justification for our attention seeking cravenness, a smokescreen for our insecurities. We claim to play to entertain others, but more likely to distract ourselves from duty. Most of us are limp imitators of the rare greats and even the greats have feet of clay. They too are deeply afflicted.

So come on, let's go.

DAY 1, Cincinnati/Columbus, OH

I look down from the Airbus drifting gently over the wooded hills of what's presumably Ohio. The landscape is laced with worming Interstates and the meandering Ohio River, flags of white smoke flaring from a power station's chimneys, sandy farmland lining the banks. The ill-gotten gains of imperialism are written on the face of this country like a palimpsest. Paradise erased, replaced by rapacious consumption, riches and inequality beyond political control, poisons leeching every-where, a sleeping gas of denial and bravado – *nothing's wrong, nothing's wrong* – suicide dressed as feverish productivity. America! Alive like nowhere else. Everything is hustle – seek success, make your stash – cash, graft, and reward. Planes tossed about like javelins from state to state feeding its vast engine, spiking the rage of trade in its blood. Onto a flight, into a car, onto the Interstate. Make friends, make a million, make it in America.

We float over a verdant suburbia studded with sapphire swimming pools and drop into Cincinnati Airport, where we are to interface with the tour bus. The touring party are a little tattered after a delayed flight from Heathrow stranded us in Philadelphia for a night. We also had hassle at customs about coming into the US with our guitars. To this we are unaccustomed, but squirm through with rube-like innocence and some arse-tightening attempts at charm, the name of our US radio hit, 'Roll to Me' twice sheepishly invoked. The officials finally wave us through with a DTR. 'Down the road', apparently. They were fucking with us, as is their custom.

I watch the bags unloaded on the apron. Our guitars travel in pairs within golf bags. Another bag, containing actual golf clubs, gets tossed on top of ours. Ouch. We drag them from the carousel, a short wheel to the bus where I insert my body into my top bunk, all dark wood veneer and fake-tan faux leather, like a gentleman's club for Costa-Del-Crime bounders. I'm in Max Bygraves' coffin. The bus trundles out and into the great shining world. We're gleaming in the Ohio sun, on the road, on the run.

The Columbus venue is a mini shed and, from the crashing over-head death rays, there is no escape. The stage at soundcheck is frying with fury. We daub ourselves with high-factor block, appearing caked in chalk. We're unused to being bottom of the bill, so we're edgy, and this and the heat has instilled a low-level panic – trying to get every-thing done on schedule and not treading on anyone's toes. There is no palpable diminishing of the heat at showtime as we clumsily stumble about, jet-lagged and glistening like guilty suspects.

There's a decent enough smattering of fans in attendance and they greet us like long-lost cousins at the merch tent where Iain and I sign T-shirts afterwards. They have the unembarrassed enthusiasm of Midwesterners, an irresistible mix of positivity and homespun hos-pitality. A woman tells me she's had a catastrophic fortnight and we have been a welcome tonic. It's neither the time nor the temperature to enquire further. We shake a lot of hands and lean in awkwardly for rushed photographs, our dubious attempts at beaming smiles coming over as people in a bit of pain.

We take a look at second act, Semisonic – laid back and melodious – but are forced by the pressures of the heat and folk with phone cameras to take refuge in the refrigerated climes of the tour bus. I'm not yet in the groove, still to figure out the best system that works between bus and dressing room. My pills wear off around nine and I sit mildly stupefied until half ten, before retiring to my bunk. I'm asleep in seconds, the grinding air-con muffled by the music in my noise-cancelling headphones. A woman's voice wakes me up with a start and I let out a small screech. I switch to an audiobook, *The Looming Tower*,* and doze off to tales of torture and religious madness.

DAY 2, Cincinnati

It's 10 a.m. and we're back in Cincinnati, parked inside the venue compound. I load my backpack and go backstage for a shower, drying myself with paper towels from a dispenser by the sink. I stroll out offsite and pay ten bucks to access an arts and crafts fair set up on the venue's periphery. It's a sea of dreadful tat: leather goods, tie-dyed rags and truly repugnant artwork. It's heaving with bovine white flesh, ambling about in a retail daze. I sit under an oak and gaze at the river, half-boiled in my denim. One good thing: tonight's shed is covered. But the heat is still fierce, its prison walls all around you, inches from your skin.

A harmony group start up from an open-sided enclosure, warbling a countrified *Have You Ever Seen the Rain?* Not today, chaps, no. Over

---

* *The Looming Tower: Al-Qaeda's Road to 9/11* by Lawrence Wright.

my shoulder, I spot a lurid portrait of Elton John rendered in violent puce and electric blue. Jimi Hendrix and Willie Nelson hang beside him, equally disfigured. The band treble and birds sing. The man sharing my picnic bench is speaking in the broad twang of the South and I recall someone telling me that Cincinnati – situated in Ohio but on the Kentucky border – has a dual personality: half Yankee, half Confederate. There are ants and red spider mites crawling through my leg hair and I go down to the riverbank where two large geese guard three fluffy yellow chicks. A red speedboat bumps past and the sun drills down as the boat's wake laps at the rocks with surprising violence. Seven waves, then silence. The geese take to the water honking a message I cannot fathom. Black spiders judder about at my feet as cotton-tufted seeds stream by on the breeze looking for somewhere to take root. I check out the band – mandolin, guitar and bass fiddle with a distinctly White Christian vibe – but shade is in short supply, so I go looking for the first food of the day. My morning pill has taken hold, so I'm alive for a few hours, the lowering proximity of the Ghastly Affliction held temporarily at bay. Make hay, make hay.

As I wend my way back to Bus World, I search for a hat. I need something straw with a wide brim. All I see are trinkets and future landfill disguised as objets d'art. I weave through baseball-hatted men slurping beer from plastic beakers, their wives in dime-store shorts and T's, ponytails threaded through white sun visors. It's an army of consumption. Bored and dazed, killing time.

DAY 3, Toledo, OH

I peek out from the tour bus window at 7 a.m., spying attractive 1930s brickwork, deluding myself we're in civilisation. We're not. The gig is in a zoo, miles out of town. Having performed in brothels, car parks, museums, shopping malls, cinemas and farmyards, I am not fazed by the presence of captive animals. I pass through a foyer filled with fibreglass beasts, make for the main gate and go find Toledo. I follow the map in my palm and start horsing up Broadway, past dilapidated clapboard houses along cracked and overgrown sidewalks. I march for miles in the cool bright morning, seeing nothing of interest and getting precisely nowhere. A few churches, a shuttered corner bar. Once I spot the grim little downtown skyline, I turn back and, as I retrace my steps, I re-encounter the small stuff I registered: an old lady on an old tricycle, two guys with a van, a little wheeled machine doing parking lot striping – a business I've never considered before but will forever remember whenever I'm parking in a striped lot. You need structure, right?

I take a tour of the zoo. I see otters frolicking, a sleeping snow leopard, a dusty African elephant stretching its trunk to pluck shrivelled leaves hooked to a cable suspended from an abstract metal 'tree'. The roofs of new-build houses poke out above the enclosure's brown walls. It's absurd. Exhausted Sunday parents chivvy their uninterested charges. 'Do you see the elephant?' Yes, dad, I see that bored creature perform boring tasks. A man takes a snap of his tiny daughter astride a moulded model of a boar. We, the dominators.

A rhino lies by a moat, its horn removed, armour glinting in the sun like a fucked tank. It looks like it's waiting for a quick death. *Please Mr Keeper, every day is carnage.* It opens an eye and regards me desolately. Or so I project: the fucker might be having a ball. I stare into a patch that's meant to be a yak's backyard. I see no yak, but there's a picture to let you know what you're missing. A meerkat perches imperiously on a fake rock, its back turned to the small crowd of humans it attracts. There doesn't seem to be anything stopping it from escaping to more private environs, but home is home, especially if you've developed Stockholm syndrome. The crowd moves on and I sit gazing at its robotic little movements. It resembles a security camera fitted with a motion detector.

Next door, beyond thick glass, there is a pair of enormous bears. Kodiak, the sign says. They have shaggy red coats and dutifully play-fight in their pool. I had no idea bears came in such sizes. These guys are like horses. In the reptile house, a frilled lizard eyes me intelligently, judgementally. There are Galapagos tortoises sitting in a pit, still as flagstones. Darwin and the *Beagle* come to mind, that phenomenal adventure that changed human understanding. We primates shuffle about and gawp.

There's a bit of sport to be had trying to spot the critters in their cases. I find an iguana hiding at the top of its tree, out of sight unless you crane your neck. A blood python lies under a pile of dead leaves, only the tip of its tail visible. Sneaky bastard. A cute little Aruba Island rattlesnake rests its chin on the windowsill like a daydreaming poet. The crested basilisk takes a bit of effort, but with patience I locate it behind a plant, green as jade and magnificently dressed in fins and frills. The king cobra lies curled in the corner of its room, cast-off skin strewn about like discarded party frocks. Everyone's ignoring the black-breasted leaf turtle and I feel terribly sorry for her. She's a pretty little thing, very tastefully attired in white, bronze and yellow. She looks profoundly sad about her kind being currently hunted to extinction. A gorgeous tree skink claws at the glass trying to break the wall that separates its prison from the universe. Before I leave, I see a poison frog and its imitator neighbour both luridly advertising danger in shocking orange. The one they use for arrow tips is red and black. Red for danger, black for death. Smart branding, like a Danzig T-shirt.

Later on, I tour round the bird bits. Of all the animals, they seem the most disturbed. The penguins stand around looking paranoid, the vultures appear deeply troubled and the flamingos exhibit an embittered unrest. Local birds flit in and out of the cages with impunity, making the exotic captives mad with envy. People push their offspring around the paths in tented carts. I stop at the perimeter and regard the suburban houses. I wonder what strange cries of anguish they hear at night. Semisonic strike up a soundcheck song from the arena and I remind myself I'm working. It's been a slow Sunday so far.

DAY 4, Indianapolis, IN

A town, a city, an urban metropolis! I crawl out of my bunk haunted by dreams of war and rehearsing in a nursing home. I was mistaken as an inmate. The streets around the HI-FI, the club in Indianapolis where we headline tonight, are of the charming, brick-built gentrified sort you now find on the edge of most US downtowns. Record shops, craft beer taprooms, gay dog walkers. There's a woman on the corner with her worldly goods in a plastic shopping cart. I give her a look to check if she wants some cash, but she's oblivious. A man further down Virginia Street is growling at a window, possibly at his own reflection.

Gavin is restless today, doing the undulating tremble that makes you feel feeble. Working my phone will be tricky for an hour until medication time. I have to schedule the pills so I'm not coming down mid-gig. I'm constantly fretting over my watch, counting out five-hour slots like a weirdly fastidious addict. But this is a piece of cake compared to the difficulties I was experiencing on tour pre-medication when I felt like a shuffling ghost locked in a dream surrounded by mortals who appeared to be living life at twice my speed.

Pre-diagnosis was even worse. I was mystified as to why I couldn't play our oldest hit, 'Nothing Ever Happens', on the guitar. No amount of practice improved my clumsy attempt to play in 6/8, a rhythm for which I'd always had a natural facility. It was weird. It felt like a mental block. I assumed it was some deep-rooted fear, an anxiety disorder which I could talk myself out of. But it persisted and, by the end of our post-Covid headline tour in 2021, I knew something was very wrong. As the gigs went by, my bass playing, a crude thing at the best of times, seemed to degenerate. I waited for the usual ease and tightness with the drums to kick in after six or seven shows, but it didn't happen. Everything got more difficult, not less. I thought I was going mad. I thought age had captured me. I thought I was past it. I booked a doctor's appointment as soon as I got back. He did the same simple tests I now do annually – some pat-a-cake action, some foot tapping – and we looked at one another. We both knew.

I go to a brunch place called Milktooth, full of thirty-somethings, career types in short sleeves and sunglasses. Angular electric guitar floats on the clement breeze, birds chatter, people spout their spiel. It all reeks of the casual success that comes with privilege and I seem to fit right in. My ham and egg bap and black coffee come to $23.15. I guess it keeps the riff-raff out. The service is rapid and invisible, the busboys Mexican, the waitresses white. Every car in the lot is a 4×4. You need the extra traction to drive over poor people. As I exit, the Doors are singing 'Don't you love her madly', followed by the Stones' 'Gimme Shelter'. It's the counterfeit counterculture.

I make for the tall buildings and come to Monument Circle, a strangely European-looking plaza with a hideous limestone column centrepiece festooned with bronze depictions of pioneering exploits. It looks like a neo-fascist lighthouse and is surrounded by enormous lampposts also cast in bronze so gaudy they're laughable. The national anthem strikes up from somewhere and I notice it's midday. I come across a small, polite demonstration of journalists protesting cutbacks. They're wearing red and they have a megaphone. What do we want?

A fair contract. When do we wannit? Oh, you know, whenever you can manage...

Tonight's stage is set up in the venue parking lot. The dressing room is a suite of voluminous rooms at the top of a staircase where you might expect to find Sam Spade's office. It's furnished with huge leather armchairs, pool, fussball, ping pong tables and a Space Invaders arcade machine. Paradise for a bored eleven-year-old boy who was born in the '60s. I stretch on a sofa but, sensing the creep of sleep, I have a coffee in a vinyl emporium opposite the gig. They have a turn-table behind the lunch counter and a little wooden stand that displays the current record's sleeve. The girl plays a rather pitchy album by War which emanates from lamp-shaped speakers hanging on cables from the ceiling. I notice they have a small stage in a corner, a quarter moon with black and white tiling and red velvet drapes, David Lynch-style. The two baby hipsters working here witter on to one another about cool stuff, attempting to establish a rapport. They'll never be friends. He's dull and plain while she's armour-plated with stainless steel. The War album wobbles to the end of side one and I take my leave. Later, just before the show, I find myself being photographed by the guy from the record store with two young men who've driven five hours from Michigan to see us. Their dad got them into us. I now see that the record guy is just shy and really quite charismatic. The night brings fresh perspective.

After the gig, a *Curb Your Enthusiasm* scenario arises. I'd earlier accepted a gift from a fan called Gerry, comprising of two bags stuffed with guitar picks branded with various Dels imagery. I leave them on a table in the bus, forgetting to tell anyone about them. Iain, discovering Gerry's gift and assuming it is newly delivered merchandise, passes the package onto Doug, our swag guy who proceeds to sell the contents along with our T-shirts. Gerry meanwhile sees his gift priced up and on display a few hours after generously donating it. Mercifully, we get hold of him before he leaves to explain and apologise. It would have been agonising had we figured this out after we'd left. I'd have been cringing about it for months.

DAY 5, Chicago, IL

Tuesday morning, back in the compound. I wind my watch back an hour and head off the outdoor arena site towards the Chicago skyline standing in the milky middle distance. My route takes me north along Lake Michigan's shoreline until I recognise a landmark; the old Harrison Hotel where we shot the video for 'Be My Downfall' in 1992. It's now a Travelodge, but in those days it was a dosshouse. We shot for two days on the top floor and under the neon sign on the roof. The area was pretty bleak back then. Now it's all universities and condos. In the Harrison Hotel's tiny elevator coming back up from the street, I found myself wedged between two residents, one incredibly tall, the other minute, both lit up like candles on crack, grinning like cartoon lizards. They generously invited me to a party and I politely declined. One floor was off limits because a three-week-old corpse had been recently found. The whole place smelled sweet with decomposition, the deceased's cells clinging to the fabric of the building.

I walk up Wabash under the elevated train line – it's *The French Connection*, *The Sting*, *House of Games*. American cities are cacophonous. Everything, from the hospitals to the hot dog stands, grinds and rattles with overworked air-conditioning units. Trucks, construction, sirens. The L adds another dimension, the noise a symphonic comfort as if all this living is winning. I find a sandwich bar for breakfast, but they weirdly don't sell coffee, so I'm forced into a chain next door. The charming non-binary server gives me a code for the gender-neutral restrooms and I luxuriate in its tiled privacy for a few minutes. It's more living space than a tour bus allows.

Chicago is a pleasing collision of rusting industrial infrastructure and gleaming 21st-century metropolis. The businesspeople come crowding out of their towers and march into restaurants at midday as the grafters in hi-vis break for Subs and Coke. A boss is bellowing into his phone: '...everybody between thirty-five and forty-two with CFO experience...' Tough for those 34- and 43-year-old financial wizards.

When the sun burns through, it's hot; when the cloud, thickens it's cool. Some citizens are wrapped up, most are without jackets. Lake Michigan makes things unpredictable. I use its omnipresence to the east to navigate back to the concert zone which is situated on an island off the Southside. Suddenly it starts to pour. I spot some scaffolding and shelter below before I get drenched. The app says it will last forty-seven minutes. Hmmm. I am not dressed for this. A woman in a summer dress taps at her phone under a parking garage entry. Those wrapped-up folk knew what was coming. I don't even have a hat, let alone a waterproof. I perch on a scaffolding pole for a bit. There are five of us under here. A line of girls file by in Eagle Scout uniforms. Fully prepared, the smug gits. It eases off and I peek through glass doors into a closed Union Station, recognising the interior Great Hall from *The Untouchables*. Turning east, I cross into Grant Park on the lakeshore, wandering across a vast deserted field of public baseball pitches. I look back at the Harrison, the Essex and the *Ebony* magazine buildings. The heat is mounting once more. I sit on some stone steps and daydream in the tranquillity unique to the big city park.

Before re-entering Jail Jolly after my day release, I take a swift turn about the vast Field Museum adjacent to the venue. Room after room of dismal taxidermy, depressing dioramas and dimly lit cases of dull artefacts for the bargain price of twenty-eight bucks. I toy with asking for my money back on the grounds that it's so rubbish that I need a drink and could be reasonably pissed on that money.

Later, I sit high up in the bleachers watching the Barenaked Ladies' crew ready the stage. The Chicago skyline stands beyond, a glittering forest. Big screens on both sides of the stage show adverts for vodka and Fender guitars. How vulgar. The wind blows the sound around. The hubbub from the waiting crowd below sounds like the clatter of gannets. No one seems too excited. We're all too long in the tooth. We know what happens. We watch this shit and go home and pretend we've enjoyed ourselves. We did once; now it's just habit.

DAY 6, Milwaukee, WI

I awake from an atrocious nightmare involving accidental deaths on a hillside for which I am suddenly a chief suspect. It's 6 a.m. and I take a piss. Strangely, as soon as I fall asleep again, I re-enter the nightmare at the same place I'd left it on waking. This is a new phenomenon. The oddest thing about the Ghastly Affliction is it randomly tossing roadblocks in your path in the form of new, often fleeting symptoms. For a while, I kept sensing people standing in my peripheral vision. I would turn to find no one there. I learned to ignore this at the cost of general spatial awareness. I now have to ask Iain not to hang behind me onstage when I'm at the mic because I have to focus straight ahead or I'll lose concentration.

Some symptoms arrive and you expect them to stay forever when they suddenly up and leave. I was dizzy for nearly a year. Not giddy dizzy, not vertigo dizzy, just dizzy, like there's a slow-motion hurricane rotating within the ocean of your head. It wasn't particularly unpleasant, just a bit distracting. I've spoken to a fellow sufferer who told me that, for some reason, she sometimes freezes going through doorways. I've not had that, but I kind of understand it. Nowadays, if I forget a pill, I'm quickly reminded by the nosedive of energy and engagement with the world that the lack of meds brings on. You find yourself perfectly attuned to a social situation, then suddenly treading water in a murk of sensory limbo. One minute you're holding court, the next you're clutching straws.

I'm up and running off the Milwaukee lakeside shed site around 9 a.m. and am in a posh café in a revamped warehouse neighbourhood by 9.30, scoffing veggie hash and grapefruit juice before horsing the half-hour to the art museum to meet my friend Bobby. Bobby was one of our hosts on our mad 1986 tour of the US when, penniless and without a record deal, we managed to persuade various fans of our first record (who had written to our fanclub) to put on little shows and put us up, usually in their incredibly understanding parents' homes. It became the making of us and we feel forever indebted to those amazing people. Bobby and I walk and talk in the pleasant building, sidling into the occasional painting that wins our attention. I particularly love Gabriele Münter's *Portrait of a Young Woman* from 1909 and there's some wonderful stuff from Haiti. A man asks us if we speak German. Bobby says, 'nein'. I ask the man if he speaks German and it's suddenly funny to us all. Plenty of Germans came to Wisconsin. I notice the show caterers are serving cheese and beer sauce.

Bobby has an appointment at noon, so I don't spend as much time as the collection obviously deserves. He writes for an online paper here and I accompany him to a pretty Lutheran church where they are holding a ground-breaking ceremony to celebrate the raising of the initial couple of million dollars for restoration work to begin. Various Christian types make short speeches on the church steps where a homeless man was murdered by a mentally ill assailant from the victim's nearby hostel. The work is to help expand the church's community outreach mental health and food programmes.

After the formalities, a few of us walk down to the undercroft, dipping our heads under aircon ducts to a safe, unopened for fifty years and for which the combination has recently been discovered. There's mild excitement in the air as Bobby fiddles with the ancient dial, finally getting the code right and opening the thick metal door. Inside is another little cupboard containing files and paperwork unseen for decades. There's also a safe deposit key. Everyone speculates humorously about the possibilities. But the further three million required to complete the building work is not in evidence. It's weird to be surrounded by these quiet people of faith in the middle of a rock tour. I sense Gavin trembling in the awkwardness and I try to smother him in a pocket, lest some minister think I've come here for a miracle. Gavin is such a faithless bastard. Gavin is a giveaway.

Back at the venue, there are plans afoot to unite all three bands for a finale and a scratch rehearsal erupts, which I watch from the back of the arena. Kris and Iain are gamely giving it a go. I'll keep my powder dry until I get through the heavy schedule of the first few weeks. I've been fast asleep in my bunk every night around the time of the final encore, anyway. I can't keep my eyes open past ten.

The Milwaukee gig is chilly and Gavin is dancing about of his own volition. On one song, which I sing without the armour of an instrument, I have trouble steadying the microphone at my lips with my right hand. I wonder what this looks like to the audience. Do they think I'm nervous? Do they think I'm a bit frail? Drunk? If I grab Gavin with my left hand, I can strangle the fucker, but it feels unnatural. Perhaps, like Ian Curtis's frenzied dancing echoed his epileptic seizures, I could make it part of the act. But I long to be normal. I don't want to have some handicap taken into account. I just want to be judged for getting the songs across, for putting some feeling over. Easier said than done when you're spending half your energy fighting the feebleness and wondering what further little errors will creep up next. A missed beat, a missed note, a fumbled syllable. I'm coming full circle. I'm turning back into the amateur I was at sixteen. Third on the bill again. Will I soon be back to being a bedroom balladeer, never to be seen on stage again, a rickety old rock singer rotting in the attic? Not if the marvellous medications keep doing their sweet job.

DAY 7, St Cloud, MN

I'm sitting outside a Mexican restaurant in Minnesota reading the *New York Review of Books*. It's 26 degrees and I'm a mile from the Mississippi. The fish tacos have cheered me significantly and I sip Coke from a big red plastic tumbler under a Dos Equis-branded sunshade. I read '*asevrec*' through the fabric. Silly mariachi music pipes from a wall-mounted speaker behind me as desultory traffic slowly hushes past. I'm in downtown St Cloud on our first day off. I'm looking onto two- and three-storey brick buildings typical of the West and Midwest around the late nineteenth century. I think they're lovely, discreetly detailed and solidly unpretentious. Not grand but honest and dependable. Wide tree-lined streets, chattering birds, brushstrokes of white across a pale blue sky. A pick-up parks up and the loud twangs of country music briefly burst out as the driver opens his door. My mariachi guys win out in the end.

I take a flight of stairs down to the river. Two companions paddle past in an old wooden kayak. How very Mark Twain. They pass under a rusted railway bridge, engineered in that Meccano style. I stop at a sign to read about the indigenous people who hunted this part of the country. There's a sad photograph of three figures sitting outside

U-shaped shelters made from carefully twined branches, regarding the camera with cold disdain. The walkway runs by a deserted office parking garage, recently built but presumably cunted by Covid. The path quickly comes to a cul-de-sac and I spot a distant circular sign on a pole denoting a Target. Might as well head there. Something to do. I'll buy a hat. And I do.

But the way is barred by roadworks. I try an improvised diversion, which looks like it's leading nowhere until I come to a set of railway tracks beyond which lies the Shangri-La of an air-conditioned super-store. I gingerly stalk over the six lines, toeing the heat-cracked sleepers like a tightrope walker. Suddenly remembering the cobra in Toledo Zoo, I steer clear of patches of dead leaves. The shop is humongous and garish and sad. I fiddle with a hat I fear might make me look like I'm trying to be a hipster sort. I decide against and go plain. Staid. That's me.

Walking back into town, I meet two bored colleagues, Iain and Brian, who are sitting roadside at a corner bar. I join them for three zero-alcohol beers which steel me for the hour and a half hike to the hotel, for which Iain accompanies me. I sense vaguely that, since my diagnosis, Iain has been keeping an eye on my general condition. It's not an unwelcome feeling, though for a time before I started medica-tion, I felt like the band were carrying me. Instead of leading, I was leaning back. The little yellow pills have corrected that. How long will they remain effective?

The sun is sliding west and north, and the evening air is pleasant on the skin. The arrow-straight route runs parallel with the Mississippi, passing detached clapboard houses that, as Iain opines, look like they could be thrown up in an afternoon. After an hour, I feel like we've decided to walk the length of the river. Maps shows seventeen days to New Orleans, but I guess that's without stopping. By my calculation (which is unreliable), you could do it in 160 days if you averaged eight miles per day.

We arrive at the truck-stop hotel around sunset. The only restaurant in the area just closed. I queue at Subway and the trucker in front of me has a holstered pistol and sheathed hunting knife displayed on his belt. He's a pot-bellied tit with a pathetic beard and a wanker's cowboy hat. His T-shirt is emblazoned with the logo, 'American Fighter'. I seethe at this exhibition of wounded, snarling masculinity. The serving staff go along making up his food as if there's nothing unusual about a customer standing two feet away boasting of his willingness, perhaps strong desire, to administer lethal force. I wonder if I just screamed 'I have a suicide vest!', he might pop a plug in my chest and scalp me for good measure. I bet he dreams of such scenarios. Fucking tool. Later, I stretch out on my big bed and stare into the black hole of the TV. Sleep comes with the stealth of a nerve agent. I'm gone.

DAY 8, Waite Park, MN

I ponce around my room, making use of the last bastion of private space for the next seven days. I dawdle over every task, basking in the unscheduled hours. We hit the venue site around noon, a shed stage with uncovered amphitheatre. I walk into the outer world, the sun lashing, my shadow so short as to be nothing at all. I find Menards, a massive hardware store, and go inside to cool down. I take a long rest on some garden furniture. A trapped bird cheeps alarm from the metal roof. I finger some work shirts and baseball caps. In the car park, men are thrusting sheets of wood into their pick-up trucks. It's a carnival of virility. I walk back to the entertainment compound.

In the dressing room, Iain and Kris are joylessly rehearsing their parts for the finale. The more I hear the song, the more I want nothing to do with it. I imagine I'll succumb to the collective positive vibes at some point, but I've not yet been awake at the appointed hour of the evening. 10 p.m. still feels like four in the morning to me. They'll be pretending to be having a rocking good time while I'm unconscious, the drone of a history of WWII audiobook clamped to my ears.

In the dressing room, I lie on a white leather sofa strewn with gold lamé scatter cushions. I'm swimming in a parody of luxury. I dab at my device disconsolately. Incoming/outgoing. Messages, messages. Through the tinted window, I see Andy perched on a stool under a sun brolly, working on his laptop. We're all just burning up the hours until action stations. This is why we used to drink and smoke weed for hours after shows. It gives your day a purpose, an endpoint to anticipate with excitement. Doing all this sober is like being forced to read your favourite books without punctuation. I bumped into a friend before coming over here. He did a lot of similar long tours on this circuit as a tech. He adopted the habit of choosing a hobby for each trip. One jaunt, he made model aeroplanes. I suppose writing this is a hobby. It certainly kills a lot of time. But so much of the time is empty of interest that it's hard to find anything to write about. I'm just throwing words into a phone. It's meaningless. It's agonisingly boring. And it's also infantilising and stupefying. We're turning into thick babies.

After tonight's show, I pop out front to meet an old friend from Minneapolis. Jodi's been diagnosed with stage-4 breast cancer. We swap commiserations. It's comforting being among people with other ghastly afflictions. You share a fatalism. Her partner is a card – drunk in that louche, pitiful but endearing way. My friend says their romance has been a thirty-year battle, but sometimes it's worth it. I hope it will be for them.

On the backstage deck, I have a conversation with Doug, our young American merch guy. He's a sweet kid with a nose for numbers.

He tells me his dad was an insurance broker with a team of a hundred salespeople. But his company was dragged under by a larger firm he was contracted to and he became sick and died. Poor guy. You can see the drive in his eyes, the hunger. I accidentally activate the microphone in my notes app and our conversation is transliterated into a long screed of garbled syntax that looks like modernist prose. I go back to the bus and listen to some relaxing Krautrock, the first Neu! album. I guess without Neu!, you don't get Wire. And without Wire, you don't get Blur. What did Blur beget?

Iain arrives in the bus back lounge having done his duty on the finale. I feel like one of those burnouts delegating more and more responsibility to others. My fire is slowly going out. Let it all die.

DAY 9, Mankato, MN

I wake up on the edge of Mantako by the Minnesota River and walk up to the main street that runs parallel with it. There are those quaint little turn-of-the-century brick edifices again. It's Saturday, hot and muggy, and there's an art fair on one of the side streets. I already know the score, but I take a look through some sense of duty. Forty little gazebos flogging objects of NO DISCERNIBLE INTEREST OR VALUE AT ALL. Just because you made this shit in your garage doesn't make it any less a candidate for instant landfill than a plastic toy made in Taiwan. The only possible reason I can see why anyone would buy this stuff is sheer pity for the artisans themselves. Don't fucking encourage them. They're deluded idiots. Stop this madness now!

I pass the university campus where graduates and their guests are flocking in a grassy square. This is one of those bastions of liberalism in a deeply conservative area. Most people look like farmers but are sporting rainbow tattoos and daring amounts of black clothing. A lot of migrants from New England, apparently. I plan my day. The Champions League final kicks off at 2 p.m. and I believe Brian has access to a feed on his tablet. I shall finish my coffee in this local gaff, swing by a drugstore for no reason at all and wend my woke way back to the happy-camper showground.

The video feed proves, perhaps predictably, somewhat glitchy. We watch the match in ten-second snippets between freeze frames, but find a way to enjoy it. Anything to break the day-long tedium. Today's venue is a smaller version of yesterday's. We change the set to avoid feeling stuck in an endlessly repeating vortex of hell. I sit out front and watch the crew setting up. Kris is strumming a silent guitar in his shitkicker straw hat. Our French-Canadian monitor guy, François, plays a cheesy ballad on our piano. It feels like it might rain, a cool breeze is mingling through the warm air. I amble down to the stage.

In the two hours between soundcheck and showtime, the weather has taken a decided turn. The wind is up, the sky grey and fat drops of lukewarm rain are smacking the plastic sheeting hurriedly employed to cover the backline. We're not sure if we'll get a green light, but we get the signal at ten minutes to go. We ply our trade to the groupings of fans dotted about the place. It all could be so much worse. I catch a song of Semisonic's set from the back of a wing, then wander off site to sit under the roof of a nearby picnic area. I can hear the crude choir of the crowd singing the chorus of Semisonic's 'Closing Time'. The green river oozes past in the gloaming. A crack of blue opens in the east. It's all going to be alright, isn't it?

DAY 10, Kansas City

At last, a long drive. I hop down from my top bunk and peek out at a loading dock under gunship-grey cloud. I've checked Maps and we're too far from town, so I walk to the nearest grocery through the undulating parkland that surrounds the Starlight Theater. I head uphill to a curious building redolent of an old Katharine Hepburn movie. It turns out to be a golf clubhouse erected in the 1900s. It has columns and towers made from flat blocks of limestone and must have been a fancy destination in the Roaring Twenties. I can see the rich folk in my mind's eye in their tweed plus-fours and brogues, caddies humping bags of wooden clubs, cigars in the players' mouths like vulgar gentry.

I stop into a local grocery – I'm the only white guy around. A young woman outside greets me welcomingly and I buy some pork rinds and sweet tea. I place my grocery bag down on a bench by a bus stop and sit and daydream for a while, the gentle breeze carrying spots of rain a balm. I popped a melatonin in the middle of the night so I'm groggy but relaxed, my heart beating sluggishly as if cased in mud. I've stuck a nicotine patch on my arm to perk myself up. There's a little white church opposite with a small needle for a spire. Cars growl by, tyres sizzling on the pale tarmac. As I turn to leave, I see an old man exiting the store dressed to the nines in checked beige suit and Panama hat, perhaps en route to church. I saunter across the open grass back to the venue, everything in rich shades of green, trees on the horizon, a thin, guyed mast reaching into the canopy of smoky cloud. The grass is long and rich with purple clover. A distant figure strolls slowly toward me like a walker whose dog has recently died.

The venue is a large outdoor arena with a huge stage built into four elaborate brick towers, topped with swooping copper roofs. It's a late '40s kind of rococo monstrosity but beautifully constructed. The site feels like the playground of a twisted billionaire with its fountains and ivy and filigree ironwork. It is a world of weird.

After soundcheck, I sit out front watching the various ushers and security staff take their positions. Some in black, some in pale blue, all in khaki slacks or skirts. The screens on either side of the stage advertise forthcoming concerts. A *Jagged Little Pill* musical, a Beatles tribute show dedicated to *Abbey Road* and the *Let It Be* rooftop performance. Rock as family entertainment drained of all context, nuance and fury.

I catch a glimpse of myself in a mirror on the bus. I can see I'm slowly going native. The baseball cap is a start. I might get some wrap-around mirror shades, Americanise my facial hair and, finally, get a mullet. The full transformation. I watch the whole show after we've done our forty minutes, including the BNL finale with Iain and Kris. The rest of us are very proud of them. They look cool up there. I feel a distant pang of jealousy, but it's overpowered by a complete inability to find a way into the Steve Miller song they've chosen. I don't see what I could add to it. Iain is doing a sterling job anyway. I might get away with remaining gloriously aloof. The Ghastly Affliction also makes learning new things hard. I'd have to listen to it for a week and that's not a thing I'd relish.

We leave around midnight for our headline day in Denver. I'm looking forward to being at the centre of things. From bottom of the heap to top of the pack. We rumble on.

DAY 11, Denver, CO

Ah, Denver! Named after the famous omelette, which in turn was named after the famous easy listening survivalist. We were here when the Timothy McVeigh verdict came in and again a few months later when Lady Spencer died. We came offstage and onto the bus to be told by our tour manager the posh royal woman was in hospital following a car crash. By the time we'd finished the encore, she had been pronounced dead. A strange atmosphere suddenly engulfed the touring party as we realised nearly half of the bus was visibly upset, the rest just confused as to why we should feel anything at all. It became so fractious that I called for a minute's silence in respect to all the dead, including the driver. That did the trick. I got drunk and phoned my father at seven in the morning from a booth in the hotel lobby. I wanted to know why this event had affected me when I was brought up to be an anti-monarchist. He had a very sensible explanation. He said, these figures are forced down your throat all your life as your tribal leaders. The monarch is on the money, the stamps, the post boxes. The monarch leads you into war. Their children and their spouses are continually held up as your betters in the media. It's wall-to-wall indoctrination. This made me feel a lot better. When I phoned my mother, she said, 'Don't be stupid. Who cares? The silly cow died because those toffs never wear seatbelts.'

I'm up at nine and off to a smug hip diner for some admittedly fine huevos rancheros. They're playing New Order stupidly loud. I buy a green shirt in a tiny vintage den and notice a very threatening sky looming over half of the city. I take shelter on the bus and wait for venue access. The Ghastly Affliction is behaving itself today for no reason I can fathom. The weird symptoms come and go as they please, no matter what you do, eat or how you sleep. It's a little over-dramatic, but sometimes the trembling feels like an attack. Like heart or panic attacks, the shaking comes upon you with such inexplicable suddenness you cast around for an assailant. I mean, I know it's stress, but without negative symptoms, what is stress but excitement? I hate that what arouses my adrenaline is so nakedly displayed. Looking forward to the pub? There goes Gavin. Reaching for a high note while making a tricky chord change on the guitar? Durraaannngg! Gavin has awoken. Watching football is amusing. All will be perfectly fine until my team approaches goal with intent and Gavin starts rattling like a pneumatic drill. In some ways, it's an education on exactly what gets your stress hormones pumping. Sex is unthinkable.

After the downpour, I walk a block north to a park, past pretty houses with porches and flags of many allegiances. People here seem compelled to display their credo, perhaps as a counterweight to all those never-questioned Stars and Stripes. The park has a lake with a central fountain. There are some big stork-like things paddling about. It's cool and green and could be any June day in Scotland. What I surmise to be bluebirds flit between trees, fleet and sleek. A private jet screams under the clouds. The rain starts up again.

The load-in is absurd. Our bus has to be parked two blocks away to plug into shore power (some call it land power), so we have to push and carry all the bits down back lanes and over kerbs to get it all from bus to venue. It's a sweatbox theatre opened in 1912, going on to be a flea-pit porn cinema in the '70s before being converted into a music venue in the mid-'90s. The dressing room lies in the basement at the bottom of a precipitously steep flight of worn wooden stairs. We played Denver a year ago, so Iain and I spend an hour trying to wrangle the set into a plausible new order replacing a few numbers with new things. It looks like a dog's dinner. Hopefully these curs will be hungry.

DAY 12, Red Rocks, Denver, CO

The Bluebird Theatre show is a hoot, the Monday night crowd galvanised by the Denver Nuggets basketball team winning a major final fifteen minutes before we go on. From our basement dressing room, we hear a huge roar go up and I run up the stairs to see what's afoot. I'd imagined Buddy from our backline crew had done something entertaining, but it was the good news spreading like laughing gas around the room. I'd forgotten what great audiences we've always had here.

In the morning, we take the short ride to the spectacular Red Rocks Amphitheatre, all sandstone slabs and scrubby trees. It's like a scene from *The Flintstones*. I hop off the bus and go into the gift shop called, naturally, Red Rocks Trading Post. Even in the wilderness, everything looks ersatz. They're flogging branded hoodies and sweatshirts, baseball caps and coffee flasks. There's a mini museum with Joe Walsh and Dan Fogelberg exhibits and a wall of crummy '70s recording gear behind glass. Tourists sleepwalk about. It's chilly, like an April afternoon in Aberdeen. We crossload our gear from the bus to a van that hauls it up the steep hill to the stage. The air is fresh and still as if in an outdoor cathedral. I take a snap of a hideous statue depicting John Denver, guitar slung across his back and an enormous eagle, wings spread, perched on his left forearm. It's repulsive and hilarious.

On the way up the steep steps to the venue, I stop at a sign listing the many restrictions and bylaws. A breathless septuagenarian on his way down gives me the lowdown. 'The museum is closed and some of the trails are roped off due to a performance, but you can get a good feel of the place.' He's lovely and I want to take him home. I thank him and we wheeze off on our separate trajectories. I wonder how Chris, our stand-in tour manager and sound man, will cope. He's not the fittest. Then again, neither am I, am I? The place is as spectacular as so many have told us over the years. The backstage area is built into the rock, like the Batcave. I sit with a weak coffee and regard the crew. Mostly in their sixties, black-clad and grizzled, they mutter greetings and swap local information. I eat lunch with our driver, CJ. He's from a Pennsylvanian Mennonite background and his great grandparents left the faith to become coal miners. CJ is now a Lutheran. I tell him about my Milwaukee church experience. He looks a bit bemused. It's not much of a story.

In 1970, when I was five, my parents took my sisters and I on a camping trip to Turkey. They drove our secondhand Land Rover through Germany, Czechoslovakia, Romania and Bulgaria. All I remember about Turkey was the Roman amphitheatres, mountain goats and the pungent aroma of my mother's exotic cigarettes, lit by my father and passed to her while she drove. This place reminds me of those spaces, built into a natural shell shape with beautiful views beyond the platform. In Turkey, it was the Aegean. At Red Rocks, it's the battalion towers of Denver's downtown. I'm looking across a timespan of fifty years and I can feel the sweetest traces of that little boy inside me. Sometimes I like him very much. But often I see he was probably a right little cunt.

Everyone is walking around looking stunned by the location. I look at photographs on the corridor walls under the stage. It looks like they must have dynamited through the cliffs and built a narrow-gauge railway to bring up the materials. In one shot from 1941, a crowd of bigwigs in panamas and fedoras stand among workers in flat caps inspecting progress. Who among them if any is still breathing? When will we too be shades?

I put a small batch of laundry in a machine. The utility room here has two attendants. The whole place is lavishly equipped with every amenity. I don't need clean clothes, but it's something to occupy my time. You spend your days sitting doing nothing, then amble off to another zone to sit and do nothing. Gavin trembles at my side, an almost welcome companion. I might be Gavin's comfort animal. I go where he goes. I soothe him to sleep. When he gets excited, I hold him firmly in my left hand.

I take the precipitous stairway down to the bus with my two little polythene bags of washing. A security guard pulls a barrier ajar to make way for me. I apologise. 'No problem, my man. Triple A. You got a God pass.' And there it is – the privilege of wandering through the halls and walls of these historic venues without hindrance, from the attics of Victorian playhouses to the caves of a mountain stage. I'm a showbiz god in a palace from Viking mythology.

An impressive number of people turn up early for our seven o'clock slot and by the end it's looking full. It has the feel of a stadium gig where the pitch is stacked up at an angle in front of you. It feels like everyone is on or above your eyeline. It's a great sound – big but fat too, and tight. I walk up the tunnel to the enclosed mixing space during BNL's set and the sound is tremendous, like a high-class PA in your living room.

I don't make it to watch the finale. I walk down the mountain for the last time to the empty bus and bunk early. We rumble out around one, leaving the miraculous Valhalla behind. I get up at five and look out over rolling plains in a smudge of dawn. We roll on, rocked to sleep.

DAY 13, Salt Lake City, UT

I spent a few minutes researching Mormon underwear yesterday at Merch Lad Doug's suggestion. I'm sitting in a pretty botanic garden, nestling up in the foothills overlooking Salt Lake City, ten yards from the bus, eyeing the gardeners and wondering if they are appropriately attired. Cool breeze, warm sun, short shadows. I notice from phone news that Cormac McCarthy has died. Lots of long shadows in those books, stretching to the desert horizon at sunset. I expect we'll see some desert soon, westbound as we currently appear to be. It's best not to look too far into the future. By later tonight, I'll know where I'll be waking tomorrow. Just now, in this garden of perfumed blooms, I have no idea.

I programme a breakfast place into Maps. The route leads me through woodland to an exit turnstile. I push through into a parking lot with spectacular views of the snow-dusted mountains surrounding the city. I walk downhill past the Museum of Natural History with its Rio Tinto wing. Nice bit of greenwashing there. In the flat valley basin in the distance, I can pick out the Tabernacle, spires pointing to heaven like a granite quiver. On the driveway from the museum, the floral central reservation is being tended to by fit young adults who look like adverts for clean Christian living. By the time I hit the highway, a gang of Mexican guys are working on the verges. It's the sort of stratification that Mormonism's founder Joseph Smith would have approved of.

I walk through the university campus to a café at the bottom of the hill. Everybody looks so super-white; culturally, sartorially, behaviourally. It's a suffocating whiteness, smiling and amiable but buttoned-up beyond belief. You feel the fear simmering beneath the well-pressed Gap apparel. An interesting family take the table beside me. Three daughters and an I-take-no-shit-looking mother, all with dark hair. The eldest has a cool Chrissie Hynde spiky do, the middle child a long beautifully combed mane and a ballet dancer's posture, and the youngest looks amazing – dark circles under her eyes and a furiously quizzical look on her face. They all speak at an imperceptible volume, almost telepathic, and come across as very serious and close. Just when I go judging Americans, along come the anomalies that prove generalisations suspect. I'm sitting in my denim and black boots. They're thinking, another of those grey-haired, boring old rock guys. Think they know everything. I know fuck all. Absolutely fuck all.

Storms are forecast and I hear low bellows of thunder from my chair on the café terrace. Rain starts up, coming down at a perfect right angle to the concrete. I head for the nearby Utah Museum of Fine Art, paying fifteen bucks to see lots of horrible oil paintings collected with no rationale or taste. On the second floor, there are some looted

Indian reliefs from the first millennium CE, all big-breasted women and pot-bellied elephant gods. The best stuff is the Mesoamerican sculpture from what is now modern-day Mexico. Bats with fat faces and weird flat human figures with pointy hats and bulbous eyeballs. Seventeen hundred years old and fresh and funny still. There's a room of twentieth-century African stuff that leaves me cold. I watch a video in the dark cube of an anteroom consisting of a seven-minute helicopter shot of the great Salt Lake. It's digitally rendered to appear like a painting and ends shortly after flying over a smoke-belching chemical plant.

Before I leave, I sit by a comforting 15-foot-tall glazed ceramic figure, *Ethnic Man* by Viola Frey. He has a red tie and his hands are clasped demurely at his waist. He's giving nothing away. He's the best thing in here. The building is very boxy with pristine hardwood floors and plate-glass balustrades. It's cool and peaceful. Distant chatter echoes from unseen halls. I weave my way out, collecting my bag from locker number 118 as I go.

The route back to the Natural History Museum takes me through Fort Douglas with its military museum on the site of an old garrison. I don't go in. Military shit makes me nervous. Who celebrates an institution whose prime function is the organisation of violence? I imagine some men find the sight of an old tank stimulating. They make me think of people on fire. The other museum up the hill affords incredible views of the valley floor and mountains beyond. I bask on its balcony, dipping a doughy cookie into an Americano. Time is tightening so I decide to do a rapid tour. The building has a clever design. A shallow gradient walkway turns slowly through the exhibits like a mountain trail. You arrive at the top floor feeling you've hardly climbed at all then shoot down the stairs to the lobby. It's like a helter-skelter in reverse – slow slide up, quick steps down. One curious element is the glass-walled fossil lab where visitors can ogle boffins at work. I watch a venerable expert unearthing a skeleton with an electric micro-chisel. Little flecks of sandstone leap into his beard. I presume the scientists detest this arrangement. It is banal to call this a human zoo, but that's precisely what it is. So I march back to Camp Merry to put myself on display. Dancing Gavin and his Amazingly Stiff Human.

After a duff show, I scarf dinner and walk through the gardens and join a trail following a river running through a small wooded gorge. I stop at a clearing and suddenly realise it's beautiful. I follow the path to a viewpoint looking over all of Salt Lake City, the lake itself shimmering in the west in the gently sinking sun. Dragonflies the size of small helicopters zip above. Crickets start to chirrup and the dim hubbub of the crowd floats up from the grass amphitheatre below me. I sit on a rock facing the sunset, dandelions the size of tennis balls shaking their seeds in the warm breeze. A bumble bee laden with pollen hovers a foot away either curious or pissed off I'm on his patch. Everything tonight is an earthly delight.

DAY 14, Nampa, ID

I squint out of the bus at midday. Parking lot, bright sunlight, everything flattened and harsh. We are in Nampa outside Boise, parked in the middle of some concrete equine metropolis, the Idaho Horse Park. Not a grassy field in sight, just some chrome trailers on the back of pick-ups. There's a sound of muffled whinnying. I'm in a denatured hellscape. Last year around here, I got filthy looks for daring to wear a mask. I pop on my baseball cap and go round the corner to a seamy thrift store filled with unwanted, mass-produced detritus. Next, to the Egg Factory for breakfast, a big soulless shed of a diner with no decor and grim black banquettes. I'm shown to a booth among ornery old coots in check work shirts and fat braces. I smear my wheat toast with livid Hammer horror gore that's so sweet it makes my heart jump. The breakfast looks bad – a grim beige arrangement – but the home-fried potatoes are really good and taste, this being Idaho, like they got pulled from the soil somewhere around here. The coffee is decent and the ketchup is Hunt's, Heinz being way too East coast for this establishment. The food is cheap, too – half the price of, say, Milwaukee.

I cross the highway to the colossal barn of a Walmart. There is a row of canoes on sale outside, rifles, tents, bras and groceries within. You could fit a mid-sized English village in here. I try on pairs of cheap sunglasses. Everything for sale is ostensibly box-fresh, but somehow looks shoddy and sad. I follow the sound of Barenaked Ed's voice back to the Fun Camp. I have essentially spent three hours touring the neighbourhood's car parks. If you like a lot, there's lots to like here.

The venue is another outdoor amphitheatre style affair, set beside Snake River Stampede, an indoor rodeo arena. I hear more neighing from somewhere. Today in the arena, they're setting up a Jehovah's Witness convention. Our route from bus to stage is a curtained-off corridor that leads round the edge of this, into the bowels of the building and out to the gig. It's very *Parallax View*. A stentorian voice intones from high in the rafters, as if God was a public safety announcer. The voice is spewing some claptrap about life in the cadences of robotic authoritarianism. It's terrifying. It's the first gig I think we've ever done where you need to ride on a golf cart to get to the stage. It's a ludicrous farrago.

On the show, the crowd don't give much back, but why should they? At one point, to no detectable response, I refer to the Jehovahs as weirdos, which is perhaps injudicious of me. I don't fancy being beaten up by a bunch of men in buzz cuts and business suits wearing name tags. I do dinner and afterwards find myself stretched out in the bus back lounge, listening to 24-bit files of *The Freewheelin' Bob Dylan* on Tidal. The guitar on 'Down the Highway' is still out of tune. Those vocal performances are still ancient and awesome.

So, thirteen shows in fourteen days. I'm holding up alright. My voice is a bit weird. It's impossible to know which frailties are just the deleterious effects of ageing and which can be ascribed to the Affliction. You find yourself turning laryngeal cartwheels to produce notes that should be easy. All I know is I feel more infirm than I think I should at fifty-eight. But I've never been this old before so how can I tell? And how will I know when it's just got embarrassing? Has it got so already?

DAY 15, Portland, OR, day off

Apart from a still-sleeping young Doug, I'm last off the bus around eleven, the clocks having gone back another hour. It's like being granted free life by God. I pack the necessaries in the bus and unpack them a minute later in the hotel. We're in the thick of the city – hip, chilled Portland. I will not scoff. This is heaven after the netherworld of Nampa yesterday.

It's a boutique hotel that was refurbished in a trendy/retro way a few years ago, but is now looking frayed at the cuffs. I walk to the Portland Outdoor Store I'd spotted a year ago (on a Sunday), so I'm excited to browse inside. On the way, I get waylaid by a hat shop. I buy cheap sunglasses and a lovely brimmed wool hat which the store owner adorns with a feather of my choice. I'm not sure I'm a feather sort of guy, but it's free and it seems rude to say no. I go native in the outdoor place, leaving with cowboy boots, a western shirt and an enormous cowboy hat. I now have two hats that I can't get on the plane home. What am I doing? Is this the impulsivity the nurse warned me about when talking me through the medication's side effects? I don't care. I am ecstatic. I am delighted. I'm a two-hat tourist. A hat twat.

I take a chair outside Grits N' Gravy and order an American breakfast. Street people congregate doing odd things. I fear the presence of fentanyl addiction; jerky, energetic movements, constant bending over double and fiddling with the contents of a bag, the same behaviour we saw in spades last year in Vancouver. At a tram stop opposite, a group are smoking from a glass pipe, either crack or meth. One of them conks out. A studenty-looking guy, about twenty-six, does manic press-ups on the sidewalk, then rolls over into the gutter silently grimacing with pain and holding his ankle. I look away and look back and he has simply evaporated. These wretched people are like mist; they drift in and out of the world without impacting it. The conked-out man comes to and goes into mild convulsions. His comrades ignore this and he keels over into an L-shape on his bench, completely sparko. It's a ragged, tragic tableau – three figures arranged like dumped refuse in the centre of a celebrated city. On the way back uphill to the hotel, I pass a man sitting in the middle of the sidewalk, fast asleep in a wheelchair. He has no feet.

So, in my overdone art deco abode, I finally squeeze out a metal splinter from the sole of my left foot that's been troubling me for weeks. When you have a condition which you know will never get better, only worse, little recoveries like this are miraculous. Seeing that minute sliver of steel ease out from my flesh fills me with enormous hope. When the man in the wheelchair wakes up, where can he find that kind of hope?

I listen to music in my lovely room for a few hours. This Is The Kit, Lucinda Williams, Sam Amidon, the Shadows. The breeze is pushing the curtain gently back and forth like a sentimental flashback in a Terrence Malick movie. This is bliss.

DAY 16, Troutdale, OR

The show is a half hour's drive from Portland in a park near Troutdale, just below the Columbia River that separates Oregon from Washington. I slope off the bus and eat a cardboard veg burger at a table in catering, listening to the bus drivers' chat about getting their buses tagged and keyed by pissed-off fans. They all bemoan artists who brand their vehicles, attracting, as it does, unwanted attention. Cops will pull them over and inspect the bus if they suspect the star is onboard. One act had a huge painting of his face on the side of all his buses and never got on one of them for the whole tour. It reminds of the time in the mid-'90s, driving through some Southern desert or other when our bus driver hollered that we were about to overtake Willie Nelson's bus. Our driver got on the CB radio and asked if Willie would give us a wave. We lined up expectantly in the front lounge and, lo and behold, the waving Willie appeared to salute us.

I meander off site, passing a small vineyard and crossing a highway to a strip of semi-wild land that looks like it serves as a campsite for the gig. In a clearing, I see raptors circling above, screeching an alarm. It's a sad sound, like a woman's scream tailing off in remorse. One bird has a fledgling in tow, swooping in to make contact, as if learning to hunt mid-air. The rapids of a busy freeway rush behind the woods and the sounds of little planes come and go above the cloud. It's cool today, fresh moisture on the wind. A couple of Mexican guys drive up in a pick-up to dump garden waste onto a pile by the side of the track. There's a red-brick hotel adjacent to the show site, converted from a grand farmhouse built in the 1910s. Inside, it resembles a Scottish country hostelry, dark wood and various bars, people milling about in that purposeless manner of the daytripper. I sit on a veranda at the side that looks onto a rich planting of firs, pines and maples. I'm in neutral gear, not yet keyed up to perform. We're on at six for half an hour. It's all a walk in the park. Something has to go very wrong.

In the heroin hour before showtime, that endless wait where one's mind considers taking up dangerous habits, I sit on a swing seat by the backstage water feature – a sunken pond full of goldfish with a grumpy-looking resident turtle. It has red stripes on the side of its face as if it's tried to apply lipstick and missed. The sun is out now and stings my skin. I rock half-heartedly and the springs squeak like ineffectual lovemaking in the bedroom next door. There won't be much rocking tonight.

Stuff does go wrong – guitars don't work. It pisses me off. But the gig's okay. People on portable chairs on a sloping lawn edged with trees. I walk around the site as Semisonic finish their set. A few people tap me on the shoulder, but they're not fans. They just want to acknowledge they recognise me, like there's a prize to be won if you spot a performer. I take a malicious pleasure in refusing to smile as I unenthusiastically shake their proffered hands. If they're not going to smile, neither am I. Am I supposed to be flattered that they know I was up there? Am I supposed to be grateful? I think I am. Fuck them. They can tell their friends I'm an asshole. It makes no difference.

DAY 17, Woodinville WA

The bus is like the *Mary Celeste*. I do a Covid test and gingerly poke around outside. Nobody about. I find the new stage manager, Sam – a lovely meek young man who exudes quiet control – and he gets me orientated. We're playing in the grounds of chi-chi winery. The very word winery raises my hackles, wherever my hackles are. The place is set in all-too-delightful gardens and is crawling with the sort of upper middle-class adult humans that make you want to wear a MAGA hat. No pick-up trucks here; strictly electric Audis. I walk away along a silvery avenue to the main drag and horse up a thickly wooded hill, trying to find some McCountryside. No luck. Every side road leads to a private residence. At an intersection at the brow of the hill, I glimpse snowy peaks, but that's the best it's going to get today. I return to the camp and shovel down awful buffet food, tepid and dry.

Wretched modern rock music appears to be playing from a white speaker discreetly set into the walls of the faux chateau outhouse that serves as the catering zone. But the speaker is mute. The music is coming from BNL's Foo Fighters-themed pinball machine that they wheel in in a flight case every day. I'm angry. I'm angry that my mother's dead, that my lover's been destroyed by a stroke, that I'm afflicted with this stupid disease. I'm angry that I've left My Love to flounder in a care home to play a thirty-minute set to a bunch of bored rich people halfway across the world for not very much money. But I'm afflicted with the drive to go on, show after show. It's all I've ever known. And without it I'm done.

This is the fear – that if I stop for too long, I'll atrophy, shrivel and freeze, unable to make the climb back to performance fitness from some short slump of indolence. Shows are the last remaining thing I can get out of bed for. But I know the disease will defeat me in time. It will simply not be possible to drag this trembling carcass onto a public stage. It's a terrifying certainty that I try not to contemplate too often. I vaguely hope to die before it gets that bad. A little plane crash, nobody else hurt, a gentle drowning. Something sudden, not grindingly sluggish and attritional like the Ghastly Affliction. And what else would I do? Even without this condition, I have no transferable skills. After the initial shock of diagnosis and the inevitable ensuing depression, I made a pact with myself that I would not dwell on the future. That place I once loved so much is now beyond the pale for me. I have no future and, even if I did, have no one to share it with. So I celebrate every show as a small victory – another one survived without catastrophe or collapse. I learn to live with the mistakes, the flat notes, the sudden judder of my plectrum, the necessary uncouth approximation of what was once, in its simple way, near perfect.

I always choose the top bunk, rear port side. It's an ingrained habit, almost superstitious. On US buses, getting into bed is a bit of a climb. You have to get your foot on the edge of a middle bunk and lever yourself up like a rock climber. It can easily go wrong. And getting out is a long drop. You suspend yourself on your elbows between the two top bunks (like a gymnast on the parallel bars) and pull your arms together over your head. Some mornings you think you'll fall forever.

The show is decent – there are a few devotees who stand and dance in the rain. The rest observe us without too much outward display of enjoyment. Afterwards, I eat and shower in the creepy lodge we're billeted in. Iain and I go to the winery boardroom to use the production Wi-Fi so we can download entertainment content in preparation for tonight's fifteen-hour bus ride. I watch *Barry Lyndon*, Kubrick's coldly cynical epic, and feel preposterously sorry for Ryan O'Neal's amoral opportunist. He's afflicted with bitter ambition and desire to regain his once-lofty status. But he's an arrogant hedonist and his resentment leads to perdition. Isn't that every rock singer career ever?

DAY 18, Cupertino, CA

I flop off the mothership around 3 p.m. after remaining in my bunk for the duration. We double drove last night, so the trip across two and a half states flew by. I throw my kit in my room and walk a mile along a highway to a burrito joint. I see from Maps we're around the corner from the great white ring of the Apple HQ. I wonder if they do tours. Here's where Steve Jobs used to have a shit etc – Graceland for tools. There's a range of hills on the horizon with the thinnest line of snow autographed on the ridge. I am forlorn today. I trudge along the traffic in the sharp light like a lost sheep. My Love calls me lambkin. I'd like to hear that today. I meander into a wine shop and stare listlessly at bottles of Californian red. I scuff into Safeway for some chocolate. There are about five customers in a shop the size of Denmark. There's a lot of mask-wearing. Back in the grey sterility of the hotel, I listen to 'Nudge It' by Sleaford Mods with Amy Taylor. An antidote of sorts.

I speak to My Love's son and he hates me. I know why. I'm lodged in America a thousand miles from those I love. I must go on. I must appear. And pretend that my heart is not broken into four pieces. They've fallen and I can't remember where I left them. My life is fucked. Fucked. Tell me now where I'm going tomorrow.

DAY 19, San Jose/Saratoga, CA

Iain and I meet our friend and original website woman, Alison, and her fiancé at 11.30 a.m. and are taken for lunch in a Silicon Valley version of an American diner. It's the exact same food you'd find off a highway in Tennessee, but five times the price. Corned-beef-hash-and-eggs-over-easy-sourdough-toast-black-coffee-no-cream-no-sugar PLEASE! Bang!

After lunch, Alison and her man Nik drive us to the Winchester Mystery House, which they explain to us was built by the heiress to the Winchester rifle company. This poor woman lost her husband and son in quick succession in the 1880s and, taking comfort in a spiritualist, was persuaded that, in order she not be haunted by their restless spirits, she must build special rooms in which these spectral entities might find peace. Or so it is claimed in typical Californian mythologising hype. On further reading, this turns out to be bollocks. We take an hour-long tour, our guide a robust young woman in period costume with some ghostliness about her countenance, through chamber after chamber. It's like wandering through the imagination of the deeply disturbed. The rooms are voids, useless spaces, full of absurd and impractical architectural features – staircases leading nowhere, windows in floors or doors opening onto walls. It's repugnant in its redundancy, its obsessive selfishness and its morbid relentlessness. As soon as we begin, I want to leave. The ceilings are low, the passageways tight and the colour scheme deeply depressing. It's like an endless tour bus with no wheels. The place drips with unprocessed grief and a kind of spoilt perseverance. It is very odd then that, six hours later, I find myself talking to Alison's friend Terry who tells me she recently lost both husband and son within six weeks of each other. I have to ask her to repeat this because I don't quite believe I've heard her correctly. How many useless rooms is she building in her mind to move through time and space?

I become suddenly tired backstage and take my leave, climbing up the mountainside to where the buses are parked above the lofty, spectacular Mountain Winery amphitheatre, built in the old Paul Masson place with its tremendous vista of Silicon Valley itself stretching from San Francisco Bay to the south. I thought the thin crowd would be too rich to care, but they respond to us vigorously and laugh along with the stupid bits. I take my last Parky pill of the day, the one that will take me through the night's last few hours to the drug of sleep, through the chambers of dreams to wake in Hollywood, where dreams go to have the living shit kicked out of them.

DAY 20, Hollywood, CA

A day off in the Roosevelt Hotel on Hollywood Boulevard, that tawdry thoroughfare where the stars' names are embedded in the sidewalk like golden gravestones, walked over like hardened, spat-out chewing gum and buffed by tourist training shoes. My corner room looks both west and north. I look down on the temporary tragedy of it. Badly dressed buffoons looking for Patrick Swayze trudge up and down outside Grauman's Chinese Theatre. The Hollywood sign hangs on its hill like a cheap choker.

Our friend from recording here in 1988, Alicia, picks Iain and I up around noon and drives us up to Pasadena where, parking by NASA's Jet Propulsion Laboratory, we hike up an arroyo through cool woods for a few blissful hours. I wear my cowboy hat and shades for the first time. I tell her my tales of woe and, like a great friend, she responds without drama. We find a dead snake on the way down which Alicia maternally carries into the grass. Her family have a corn snake at home called Dennis. It eats one live mouse per week. We go for a late lunch at an Eastern Mediterranean place in Glendale. I notice in the toilet there's a little video screen set into the top of the urinal. It's advertising holiday destinations. All I see is a drone shot of the Aral Sea with a line of piss running beneath it.

I lie on my four-poster on the ninth floor of the Roosevelt as the sun dips behind the ridge of Mount Olympus. Perhaps I'll never be in LA again. What does it matter? I'll never be well again either. I'll never be twenty-eight again. I had a nice day today. I open the window to feel the temperature. A little devil in me suggests walking round to the Frolic Room (where I was once offered crack in a toilet cubicle) and ordering a drink. But I know where the devil leads and it's not the pleasures of the past but the regrets of the future.

DAY 21, San Diego, CA

I snooze in my bunk on the short drive south from LA to San Diego and crawl back into the world around 3 p.m. to find myself on the pretty but antiseptic campus of San Diego State University. It's a meticulously arranged grid of old Spanish mission-style buildings with red tiled roofs, and smart modern brutalist-lite blocks. From the seamy toxic edge of Hollywood at night to the pristine esplanade of SDSU in the fresh afternoon, the contrast is bracing. As I explore the campus, sirens moan and a cop car, a fire truck and a couple of ambulances appear. I see someone pumping their arms on an obscured body and walk on, not wishing to rubberneck.

At the next corner, I hear some sporty kerfuffle and peer through a chain-link fence at a lacrosse match between Italy and Hong Kong China. Italy score within seconds of the start and dominate from there on in. When the players take a break, they play a Morgan Stanley advert through the PA. I take a seat on a shaded concrete bench and a lovely woman called Julie comes up to say hi. It turns out she was married to Cathal Coughlan, who died last year, and we have mutual acquaintances in Susie and Adam from the Katydids, who opened for the Dels in the late '80s. Cathal was the firebrand singer with Microdisney and Fatima Mansions. I remember admiring his lyrics and intensity at the time. In the late apartheid era, they had the good grace to name an album *We Hate You South African Bastards!*. I sign a book Julie is reading about publishing rights, having been left with a tangle of deals in her late husband's estate. I wish her luck with that. She has a tote bag emblazoned with my second solo album title. She's been in London for forty-three years and doesn't seem overly thrilled to be home. She exudes the quiet deflation of grief I seem to have encountered so much recently. It's an elegantly poised air of raw disappointment. An ambulance comes back up the way, siren on but moving at less than urgent speed.

I walk around the university, its white buildings gleaming in the clean, early-evening light, surprisingly green hills lying in the distance beyond shapely pines like a Cézanne painting with a parking lot in the foreground. I buy bananas and trail mix in a Trader Joe's and stroll around the outdoor arena where a swarm of security personnel are gathering, their red shirts printed with the word ELITE in big white letters across their backs. There are airport-style metal detectors at every entrance gate. A cool breeze comes swimming through from the nearby ocean. Gavin twitches anxiously at my side waiting for our cue. I wait and wait and wait.

DAY 22, The 'Greek', LA, CA

I walk down Vermont Avenue from the venue through shady groves and faux chateaux, those hilarious Hollywood houses that look like they're made out of cardboard, to a zone I remember well from my two months spent idling and exploring in 2008. I parked myself here at the end of my first solo tour, hoping to write and pick up gigs on the west coast. I did neither. I just drove around buying films noir on DVD to watch on my laptop at night. I wrote one song and played one gig, but I got to know east LA. My walk is juddery downhill, but the first pill kicks in and it evens out. Gavin trembles fitfully. They tell you the principal effect of dopamine depletion is an inability to concentrate on more than one thing. If I focus on my gait, I can kind of impersonate a normal person's stride. But I couldn't chew gum with an air of insouciance while doing it.

The zone I aim for near Little Armenia is unchanged. I stop into Skylight Books where the Byrds' 'Eight Miles High' is playing. As I claw out a copy of one of my favourite novels, Denis Johnson's *Train Dreams*, a man speaks behind me. 'Amazing book,' he says. I tell him I can't stop buying copies for friends. It's a comforting exchange, like meeting a fellow member of a secret society far away overseas. I buy more cheap shades and a lovely short-sleeved shirt in a corner used togs shop where they're playing a doom-laden art-film soundscape. In a diner, I order huevos rancheros which, due to a rent in the space-time continuum, arrive seconds before I've opened my mouth to order. The food is as grotesque as the preparation time is short. At a table outside, a young Korean guy is having his photograph taken. He poses with food as the snapper crouches and twists around him. When they're done, he wolfs down the leftovers. He's in distressed designer white denim and looks a willowy seventeen. His face is a ghostly mask of pale make-up. The speaker above rains Lana Del Rey. I pay the waitress, who looks like Lindsay Lohan. The sun glances off the sidewalk like a jet of diamonds. It's burning my right temple, but I'm armed with my big Portland cowboy hat. I ponder what to do next.

I amble down to the intersection at Hollywood Boulevard, all things suddenly becoming seedier – car washes, lap dancing clubs and a Goodwill thrift store full of Gap rags and H&M rot. Twenty years ago, you could still find old 1950s Californian-made suits in such places. Now it's all mass-produced fodder from the Far East, hanging limply on the rail, unused, unwanted and unfashionable, despite being made mere months ago.

As I climb back up the hill towards the Greek Theatre, the temperature drops at each crosswalk, the silvery walking-man profile calling me on. Each degree cooler, the property prices get hotter. Gavin shakes at my side as if I consider the world dubious – a bad bet – which perhaps I do. I employ my various strategies: the Prince Charles – left hand clasping right wrist behind my back – and the pocket swagger, where

I stuff the bastard into my right front pocket and swing my left arm with all the chutzpah of the fully abled. Hooking my thumbs behind the straps of my rucksack is most effective, but makes me look like a middle-aged rambler. I'm a ramblin' man.

At the top, I dump myself on a concrete picnic table in a scrawny little park. There's a kissing couple and a cadaverous sunbather laid out on the sandy lawn. This is the weird thing about LA. You're never far from an oasis of sun-dappled tranquillity and yet always less than a mile from a freeway that will take you anywhere that matters in twenty minutes. I've always said it's like someone has flattened out London with a steam roller to ten times the size, so all that's narrow has become wide and all that sticks up has been stunted.

I'm spending as much of the gig days as I can off-reservation. I don't feel like I fit in with the whole three-band collegiate atmosphere. I spend my time simpering and it's becoming a chore. Sometimes the Ghastly Affliction just renders you a little stunned. You find it impossible to think of a pleasantry or some bon mot or parting shot. You feel like a smiling goon. I don't really want to talk to anyone for that reason. I have nothing to say and no one to say it to.

The Barenakeds do soundcheck parties every day. This is where a band sell special tickets to fans who get to sit in the front row, watch the fucking soundcheck and meet the group afterwards. It's my idea of hell. It's been suggested to us several times and we've always refused to do it. There's no such thing as easy money. And if there is, you should be ashamed to take it. The digital era has made so much personal time publicly available. Every second of our time can be commodified. That's all social media is – the packaging and selling of the formerly private. And that's what THIS is too, except you can't slap a crying-with-laughter emoji at the bottom. I don't care what you think. I'm just killing time.

DAY 23, Indio, CA

Today we are on Native American land doing a casino show, the first indoor show of the tour. This is a good thing. It's 35 degrees outside. I do some music and movies downloading (for tonight's long drive to El Paso) in the dressing room of a big barn of a place before vainly wandering abroad for breakfast fare. The map leads me into a busy bowling alley full of local families madly chucking balls of hardened resin down oiled wooden lanes. The activity is feverish, as if the air-con is making us all giddy. We used to love bowling on tour, but the appeal has waned. Maybe it's the footwear. Now we all stare into our glowing devices all day, cocooned in a self-curated culture. I order a quesadilla, paying in cash just for the thrill of it. There's a broad mix of ethnicities here – I'm guessing South and East Asian, Mexican, Native and European American. Who knew what a melting pot bowling could be? TVs above the unoccupied lanes show sports and adverts. Baseball, tennis, golf and NASCAR. I think I see a promo for Sleaford Mods. I blink and realise it's a commercial for Seafood Pod. It's cacophonous and invigorating, like the inside of some giant organism's brain.

I take a gander around the outdoor part of the complex. Some kids frolic in the hotel pool braving the beating sun. There's an outdoor stage hosting tribute acts. Last night, Weezer; tonight, Social Distortion. Quite specialised. Probably all the same musicians. The stage is surrounded by cooling fans of every size, a nearby patio awning spews the fake mist of outdoor air conditioning, contributing to the warming planet while cooling precisely nobody. I come across Andy who is sitting on a bench under a tree, the only shade around. He's reading about the French Revolution and tells me about its founding compact, the Tennis Court Oath. We prattle about inequality and the historical necessity of revolutions to close the obscene distances between rich and poor.

I walk back to the gig in the baking world. This is the insane side of America – entire populations reliant on refrigerated air and water piped in from miles away. Chop off the mains and everyone's fucked. You'd have to live in a cave and drink the blood of ants. But there are no caves and the ants have all shrivelled up and died.

DAY 24, El Paso, TX

I hop out of my bunk around five and see the sun come up from behind the ridge of a range of dust-pile hills. We're crossing south Arizona en route to El Paso. The interstate passes through a wide valley of green scrub. We pass trailer parks, cattle ranches and pecan plantations. I guess if any nut can take the heat, pecans can. It's already 21 degrees and will be forty by the afternoon. We cross the state line and are in New Mexico. The landscape crowds around for a little, then opens up onto the endless miles of scrubland that cover so much of the southwest. I retreat to my bunk.

I doze 'til ten, listening to the superb last two matching-pair Kevin Morby albums, *This is a Photograph* and *More Photographs*. They share some songs in different forms and are both concepts based on an old family photo, beautifully recorded with gorgeous string arrangements. He's a Brooklyn-based Texan, but sounds very Australian to me. I schlep to our day-room hotel around the corner in mad heat to be rebuffed by a snippy blurt of a reception hipster. Plan B, breakfast. It's a Sunday morning in pretty downtown El Paso and I find sanctuary in The Unbranded Tavern – Mexican staff, friendly as fuck. My recommended veggie breakfast burrito is fantastic, the '80s rock on the sound system an apposite accompaniment. John Mellencamp,

Robert Palmer, that sort of thing. The folk in here are drinking noon-day craft beer with their food. There's a still of the three principal characters from *The Big Lebowski* above the door, three screens show-ing different sports and two framed shirts – one baseball, one soccer. One of the TVs just shows footage of people punching each other. I hunt museums in Maps, but everything is closed. Damn. I spot a vintage clothes shop that opens at 1 p.m., but that'll only kill half an hour. I sit at the counter and stare at the bottles of liquor on the gantry. Redemption, Fireball, Buffalo Trace and Dano's Dangerous Tequila. 'Careless Whisper' comes on. Dear George, the Christmas Day casualty. I hope he's having good stoned sex in the spirit world. The tavern's windows look on to a delightful city square. Kids play in a spouting water feature and a group strolls by, one member wearing a hat with brim so generous it provides shade for much of his group.

I walk out into the furnace finding myself on a tree-lined strip of two-storey buildings, their ground floor shops bursting with cheap goods in gaudy colours. I duck into Starr's Western Wear for half an hour and browse among the heavily branded synthetic shit, none of which is manufactured across the border, all of it from China. They have Stetsons in a glass case with $500 tags. Nothing to see here. I mosey back to the bus. It is too hot to stroll. Perhaps I less than mosey, my gait is more of a defeated slouch. I pass a man in classic Tex-Mex gear – cowboy hat, shirt and tie with no jacket, low slung belted suit trousers and cowboy boots. I take temporary shelter at a deserted bus stop. Birds cackle in the trees and a weathered man cycles unsteadily past with twenty plastic shopping bags hung from his handlebars.

I desire siesta in some dingy back room. The bus will have to suf-fice until these cunts at the hotel give us our day rooms. I find Buddy sitting in complete darkness onboard. The generator is off. No shel-ter here. I walk into the wank hotel on the stroke of three and am

finally bestowed with plastic key and Wi-Fi code. Thumping choons
infect the air from a pool party beside reception. Some reception.
The trouble with the high service standards in the US is you become
as enraged as an infant when it breaks down. These guys have been
struggling all day and have descended into defensive surliness causing us, the guests, to become petulant. There's a sweeping view east
from my seventh-floor roost. I sit in an upholstered swivel chair and
survey the city below. A goods train worms sluggishly through town.
I give up counting at a hundred wagons and it slows to a halt. It's now
40 degrees. I count the minutes until I can take my second pill. Nurse,
my infusion!

I read in the chilled box of my room for a few hours before I go
looking for dinner around eight. Everything is closed. I linger outside
a charmless corporate seafood restaurant before deciding to walk a
bit further in the still-suffocating heat. And there she is – The Tap!
The very bar where Stuart Nisbet, my accompanist, and I ended up
in 2014 after a night spent gallivanting around the gay area. It's a classic American bar with counter and stools down one wall and booths
lining the other. Neon beer signs, Mexican football on the TV, pool
table at the back. I remember watching a proper little jazz band rattling away at the end of the narrow room, squeezed together as if in a
transparent elevator. The place is a miracle. I order the recommended
Mexican plate Number 1 and a zero beer.

As soon as I sit down, Echo and the Bunnymen's 'The Killing
Moon' starts up from a lovely warm-sounding speaker system. Thank
you, fates of travel. I message the remaining others (three of our party
elected to fly to Austin from Indio this morning) and the four – Andy,
Jim, Buddy and Brian – arrive just as I'm leaving. They should have a
decent few hours in there before the carriage turns back into a pump-
kin at the stroke of midnight when we re-bus to overnight to Austin.

As I round the corner to the lot at the hotel's rear, I have a paranoid apparition of a vacant space where the bus should be. Abandoned by the mothership. I have held on to my room key for this (unlikely) eventuality. The heat was too much for the generator today so the bus has been stewing in the west Texas heat for twelve hours. But CJ, our trusty driver, has topped us up with coolant and we sail into the Texas night. It's still 36 degrees.

DAY 25, Austin, TX

We're on the University of Texas at Austin campus. I pack the necessary in my backpack and head for the nearest used clothes outlet. I'm on main thoroughfare Guadeloupe so am orientated. I was here for a month nine years ago, recording the worst of my four solo albums with a moody, uncommunicative producer and a bunch of uninspiring musicians who regarded themselves as some kind of supercool troupe of New Americana gunslingers – apart from the peerless David Garza, who took pity on me and cheered me up with some beautiful piano playing and Bob Dylan stories. The situation wasn't helped by the fact my father had been hospitalised with a catastrophic stroke two weeks before I was scheduled to start. I ended up staying in the guesthouse of an acquaintance of the producer, the landlady of which slipped me alcohol in a juice she'd brought me before attempting to seduce me. I had to kind of muscle her out of the door like a Jehovah's Witness. This was awkward as technically it was her door. And she was fondling my bare feet at the time. Had our relative sizes and sexes been reversed, this would have been a very dangerous and frightening scenario. As it was, it's merely an anecdote. But coercion is horrible. You simply don't know what to do.

It's 36 degrees in Austin and walking is unpleasant after ten minutes. I dive into a taco place and have eggs and spinach. It's ridiculously cheap. The students here are all lean. I imagine they're too rich to have been force-fed fast food by the system. You can see they're all destined for success. The campus is swarming with next term's freshers excitedly checking out their future. I hear a kid discussing how hot their dorm will be tonight. As a boy who went to his hometown university, I never experienced such tantalising moments of expectation. It was just more school, so I fucked off halfway through the first term to become a full-time chef. The student grant bought me a mixing desk and a Revox reel-to-reel, and the chef's wages helped pay for rehearsals. I'd signed a record deal by nineteen. I still have a bunch of textbooks I've never read. They'll need to go in a great purge. I feel one coming.

The Austin show is indoor in the sizeable Bass Concert Hall. It's Semisonic's final show, so the whole three-band entourage sidle on to do a little dance during one of their numbers. Being a lead singer, I hop up on the percussion riser to ensure I'm seen. Kevin from BNL says 'Thanks for joining us!' in a way that is both sweet and gratingly patronising. I've been successfully avoiding joining their nightly finale with the double excuse that I need voice rest and the Ghastly Affliction leaves me exhausted after I have dinner. Both excuses are truths, but I feel they'd prefer to have me involved. It's like being in second year school without a peer group – loitering at the periphery, scuffing your feet, trying to appear nonchalant. I'm fifty-eight for fuck's sake. If I don't want to do something, I don't have to feel guilty about not doing it. I'd join them if I felt I could add something but the thought just leaves me feeling dead inside. Mind you, I am dead inside. And increasingly on the outside, I think. When I see myself on video now, I look away. I look so stiff, my face frozen in a desperate rictus. I *look* afflicted.

DAY 26, Austin, TX to Tuscaloosa, AL

I'm sorry to be leaving Texas. Despite many Americans' snobbery, it's always charmed me. Folk are very gregarious and open. Austin's liberal certitudes would be insufferable outside of the context of wild, freebooting Texas. There are thirty million Texans. They're not all the stereotypical Republican, insular, gun-loving yee-ha's mocked by coastal stand-ups. Outside the theatre, I meet a guy from Belarus and a family whose matriarch is from Berlin. She prefers Texas to Berlin. Not sure I'd go that far. But if there's a frontier still in the US, it's here.

An hour out of town, our driver CJ pulls into a truck stop to introduce us to the delights of Buc-ee's, a kind of redneck superstore. We institute a quick ten-dollar-limit, most-interesting-thing-in-your-pocket competition. My weak entry is a pair of branded 'no-show' socks. Kris has 'laser finger' rings and Brian an amusing survival whistle which features a compass, thermometer and magnifying glass. Iain wins by doing a striptease to 'The Stripper' tune, revealing a truly disgusting branded crop top, but is immediately disqualified for spending over budget by four bucks. It's two in the morning. I am overjoyed to be up so late.

I pop into an empty front lounge around 8 a.m., the dry scrubland now transformed into the wooded and lush landscape of east Texas. This part of the world – Mississippi, Louisiana, Alabama, Georgia, north Florida – is a place of swamps and storms, sultry and humming with a weird erotic menace. Warm rain hangs in the atmosphere at night like base temptation. Everything is driving you mad by seduction. You want to swim in its decadence and drown in molasses.

But this is no molasses. This is Dante's inferno. As I step out of our hotel in Tuscaloosa, Alabama, I find myself wading through a toxic sludge, the wind thick and cottony like wool soup, the temperature a static thirty-six, unmitigated by the hot squally air. I bend into a coffee shop for instant relief and down an Americano before braving the walk for some late lunch. A youngish guy with a granite-coloured laptop sits opposite me and stands almost to attention when his older assignation arrives. The power imbalance is immediately blatant. The young guy simpers away, suddenly looking deadly serious when he thinks his interlocutor is making a point. It looks like a job interview or a meeting with a potentially big client. His craven deference reminds me of me when I'm with people I admire. You should see me with James Kirk, Paul Buchanan, Jim Moir or Edwyn Collins. I'm like a schoolboy sitting on Pelé's knee. It's repulsive. Edwyn dropped into a rehearsal last year. I awkwardly held the fist of his hand on his bad side in a parody of a handshake. And we played a song! 'Be My Downfall'! Why?! Why did we finish our rehearsal in front of him and his son, William? Were we still trying to audition for Postcard Records? Nonetheless, it was an unforgettable moment for us. If you find me giggling like a baby in front of you, I either want you to be my dad or know you're more talented than me. I look at the young guy in the coffee shop again. He's gazing into the old guy's eyes, hand on cheek and chin, like he's in love. It's so submissive, I want to slap him on the side of the head. You don't need this guy! He'll never pay you on time. He'll never praise you. Every son's father is a mother-fucker and everyone a motherfucker's son.

The lunch place I've selected is Rock N Roll Sushi, the menu (a repurposed Sinatra album sleeve) full of ridiculous names for repulsive combinations – British Invasion Roll, Tour Bus Roll etc. There's an awful lot of fried matter that belongs in another cuisine entirely. I opt for relatively safe standards. The music they're playing might be described as nu-punk prog. I Shazam and it's, ergh, The Offspring.

A caterwauling tower of shit. The food arrives and it looks genuinely disgusting. It has a sweaty patina like a rancid chicken. My chopstick skills are still just about extant, but when I rest my hand between mouthfuls, Gavin starts to tremble as if I'm conducting a tiny orchestra. Josh, my callow server, approaches twice to inquire how I'm getting on. Well, Josh, my mouth is full of this shit so obviously something's going in the right direction. The rock 'n' roll part of the deal in this establishment is fulfilled by atrocious '90s drudgery – Pearl Jam, Creed – all nasal guitar sounds and impassioned Kermitty warbling. Grunge was such a horrible genre. Britpop looks so fresh and fun in comparison. Mind you, so does shingles.

I encounter the others emerging from a bar where the food was filth and the cutlery filthier. They're like a search party that's forgotten what it's looking for. They forlornly walk down the single high street for further entertainment as I turn back to the hotel. It's the usual small-town, two-storey brick main street, with peach blossom trees surrounded by suburb. There is a nice former office block, from the 1920s maybe, that's been renovated and converted to apartments. It's a quiet place with ruddy great highways running through it. In the lift, a potential student here talks to an older woman. What are you majoring in? asks the elder. Marketing, replies the teenager. Oh, fuck off, I think.

I creep back out around seven, but the restaurant I navigate to is too busy and too upmarket. Casual dining only on tour. I go into a grim-looking Mexican place because it has outside seating. I ask the waiter to recommend something from the soiled laminated menu. Perhaps he thought I wanted him to recommend me something to regrout my bathroom tiles. My food is slathered in a grim white sauce. Flesh from disparate animals – some land-based, some not – cowers under this wet cement. I spoon the mixture gingerly into a flour taco.

You wouldn't feed this to Hitler's dog. Here I am again – the whiny limey. But it's cheap. As shit. Less than fifteen bucks for a substantial stomach full of calories. Bad food is cheap. And there's no earthly reason why this should be the case.

The sun has sunk and the sky, criss-crossed by power lines, is a grey-blue. Crickets have their hands firmly pressed on their electric buzzers. Someone starts up the hacking cough of a Harley. I suck Pepsi through a straw as the day gets sucked into the night.

DAY 27, Tuscaloosa, AL

At the amphitheatre around noon, I swing by catering for an insipid coffee, the room full of new faces, the lovely Semisonic having gone home to be replaced by an act called Five For Fighting. The little I know about this band does not predispose me to taking a kind view of them, but I try to contain my prejudice, hoping to be pleasantly surprised. I walk up a hill passing under a wooden railway bridge, its pillars freshly daubed with creosote. I take a side road towards a blue water tower that resembles a *War of the Worlds* invader. A 2-foot-long black snake slithers across my path. Better not step into the grass, I decide. It's the first time I've seen a snake move like that in the wild and it's much less threatening than when they're standing bolt upright looking keen to strike.

I'm on Martin Luther King Jnr Boulevard and I take a left down a street signposted Newtown Historic District. It's a neighbourhood of dilapidated clapboard houses, with some junk-strewn yards and a lot of weeds. Silicon Valley it is not. At a cul-de-sac, I see a family sitting on their porch. They're all coughing like plague victims waiting for the wagon. I nod hello and they gawp like the undead. I don't wish to take a poverty safari, so politely turn back. The heat is crashing around me like a boiling sea. A large raptor wheels above the high trees. If I were a pilgrim I'd get straight back on the ship.

Five For Fighting break into 'Bohemian Rhapsody' during their soundcheck. Deary me. At least the stage is in shadow, so it could be worse. We traipse through our check stunned by the temperature. Thick air. I'm coming down from my first pill, so pop another. I'm drug-dependent. We banter in the dressing room about taking heroin. At least it would be a hobby. Wake up, find dealer, score and fix. That'd kill most of the day. I'm doing two crosswords and three other word puzzles every day. That does an hour. But if you can't walk beyond the site, the claustrophobia and ennui begin to grind you down. Andy plays some Charles Mingus. Christ it's warm.

DAY 28, New Orleans, LA

I set controls for the museum district. The route takes me through a part of downtown I'm unfamiliar with. I'd forgotten how unique the city is – the bourbon architecture, the daytime drinking, the sopping heat drowning one's rectitude, corrupting one's moral compass. I stop into St. Patrick's on Camp St with its vaulted ceiling, busy stained glass and enormous triptych behind the altar. It's serene and cool with the required bouquet of incense. A group of congregants are muttering Hail Marys in the corner. They're repeating lines fed to them by a disembodied voice as if they're training. Suddenly my map barks out an instruction on my phone. I fumble to turn it off like a panicking fielder. I worry I'm about to make a fart noise. I must follow my voice and the believers theirs. I hop it.

First up is the Ogden Museum of Southern Art. An airy, five-floor building, you climb the sharp black staircase through eras from early nineteenth-century portraiture to contemporary video installations.

There is some nice naïve folk art and some great photography. Most of the sculpture, abstracts and landscapes are poor. I really like Clementine Hunter's *Chaleur: The Sun Gives Life to Everything* from 1962. I look her up later. Born on a plantation in 1887, the artist picked cotton from the age of eight.

I cross the street to the National WWII Museum. I've been listening to the audiobook of Antony Beevor's history as a sleep aid every night. I am constantly waking up to mass suicide, mass rape, mass execution, mass starvation, mass murder. World War II was an international orgy of violence and inhumanity that happened on a colossal scale, and at an insane speed and intensity. The numbers are terrifying. It's a horror show that has had an incalculable effect on human consciousness. And as I walk into the museum, pay my thirty bucks and melt into the crowds of sun-stupefied white tourists, assaulted on all fronts by patriotic symbols and jingoistic sloganeering – the Solomon Victory Theater, the Hall of Democracy, Campaigns of Courage, the US Freedom Pavilion – I want to leave. I should have known when I was offered a discount if I'd 'served'. This force-feeding of the lie, in both the West and former Soviet countries, that World War Two/the Great Patriotic War was about the triumph of good over evil is repugnant. It was a cataclysm of rampant opportunism, a resource war wrapped up in a race war. It was an explosion of greed, hatred and prejudice. But the story here is the same: bad (foreign) men do nasty things, the good guys prevail and everybody goes home. The place is crawling with men in buzz cuts and excited little boys peering at weapons. It should just be a big black fiery pit that enslaved soldiers throw babies into. I mean, they give you a dog tag for a ticket.

I go into Flamingo A-Go-Go for lunch round the corner because it has a leafy courtyard. But sitting outside is an error. I order a Coke and slurp it down, trying to cool myself from the oesophagus out. It's 36 degrees. David Bowie's "'Heroes'" is playing. I think of those 'heroes' from the war sacrificing their lives, often in prolonged agony and terror, to keep the factories running and the owners rich. The appallingly asymmetrical crime of it. Hundreds of millions of victims and a handful of perpetrators. And they the victors. There's an old US Army truck in the corner of the courtyard. They use it as a cupboard to store spare chairs.

After the gig, I go looking for food and try a seedy kebab shop-type place. Two skinny youths offer me coke and weed in the doorway. They appear to be using the joint as their HQ – charging their phones, slouching on the tables. The tiny Latino guy behind the counter is watching one of their number like a hawk. This guy is a bit too high and talking a little too fast and a little too loudly. There are four of these guys – all skinny, fit-looking and about nineteen. They don't seem to be turning much of a trade. Outside, the night air is like treacle. I walk past shadows slumped in doorways, bodies stretched out on the sidewalks. It's impossible to tell the living from the dead.

DAY 29, Atlanta, GA

Back to the big tent and I'm happy to be. There's a storm coming in and it feels safer with all the extra crew around. The Barenakeds' soundcheck party shuffle into the amphitheatre in the first fall of rain. The raindrops are as big as globes and explode on impact. I run the short trip from backstage to the bus and I'm drenched. There's no soundcheck today, which keeps things exciting. Our monitor engineer, François, has been exceptional and is always cheerful. It's a luxury to have him on our side. The venue is a deep bowl cut into mature forest. It's all very *A Midsummer Night's Dream*.

The rain lasts an hour and I walk up through the venue and find myself on a quiet suburban avenue. I continue uphill past enormous McMansions nestling among the beautiful canopy. These semi-palaces are designed in a neo-colonial style, some with comical home-on-the-range chimneys staggering up the structures as if self-built. But all these monstrosities have been flung up in the last few years. They look like they've only today been broken out of the blister packs they came in from the Bugs Bunny Store. The vulgar, vicious rich. These people will be the reason we can't soundcheck, despite the constant racket of cement mixers and leaf blowers.

The beguiling Semisonic are a distant memory as Five For Fighting's bombastic and patriotic pomp takes their place. I'd been introduced to the perfectly lovely John after our Tuscaloosa show. John *is* Five For Fighting, the name being a metonym for his solo singer-songwriter thing. John, according to Wikipedia, is fond of Elton John, Billy Joel and Queen – a suite of influences that couldn't be better designed to put me off. His act starts out a bit David Gray, all tremolo high notes and jaunty tempos, but descends (via a long interlude celebrating John's dedication to US troops and support of Volodymyr Zelenskyy) into sentimental balladeering, finishing on a note-by-note rendition of 'Bohemian Rhapsody'. I can honestly say it's the most horrible thing I've ever seen. It suddenly puts the whole tour in a weird place – a witty Canadian pop group and a sarcastic Scottish pub rock band bookending a big, heart-on-sleeve, profoundly patriotic American plonker. Boy does he plonk, his digital keyboard hidden inside a hollow grand piano case. We all hated his act so much that we're going to have to avoid him for the rest of the tour. How do you look into the eyes of someone whose work you respect so little and not give something away? I guess we can talk about the weather.

DAY 30, Greensboro, NC

I have my first fitful sleep of the trip. It's 2 p.m. by the time I feel I'm sufficiently rested. Never set alarms unless you have to. I find a diner on Maps near the bus, but am waylaid by an old wigwam-style IHOP that's been repurposed as a vegan fast-food outlet called Mike's. I am greeted with gracious hospitality and order the recommended Carolina burger. At first bite, I decide I've been hoodwinked. I'm supposed to avoid protein on these pills and this is obviously beef. But weirdly moist and tasty beef. I scan the menu printed above the serving counter. 100% VEGAN. ALL ITEMS AND INGREDIENTS ARE PLANT-BASED. I wonder if they count cows. I mean they are essentially plant-based. All flesh is grass, after all. Not only is this patty sandwich meaty, it's fucking magic. It's one of the best burgers I've ever eaten. There's a list of four, and two of those cost three times the price of a regular burger in a standard fast-food outlet. I give the girl my thoughts when she enquires. She asks where I'm from. Scotland, I say, where such food should be on the NHS. The clientele are mainly Black and the music is good. I'm coming back for dinner.

As I leave, I notice Secrets Cabaret Adult Entertainment across the parking lot. Opposite that, the Immanuel Baptist Church. It's a crossroads of civilisation. Down the main drag, I find a video/CD/vinyl emporium. As soon as I touch a (Nick Lowe) record, the ornery septuagenarian douchebag behind the counter comes out and lectures me on putting the albums back in exactly the right place. Everywhere there are signs warning not to remove records from their sleeves. These are used albums and most cost more than fifty bucks. The old bastard then goes to the door and yells at a young couple for taking the wrong parking place. I should have used the distraction to hide a Steve Forbert album in the Grand Funk Railroad section. That'd fox him.

It's exceedingly close today. A storm front is sweeping by and BNL's production guys are watching weather apps with alarm. They cut our soundcheck short to lower the stage's tarpaulin roof and cover the gear with polythene sheeting. I watch it all happen from a seat in the stalls. There is the odd fat spot of tepid rain, but the prevailing opinion is that the storm should miss us. Whatever happens, we'll leave the stage drenched in something. The amphitheatre seats are weathered green plastic and a team of women, uniformed in blue polo shirts and chino shorts, are marking seat numbers on the concrete aisles with big glow pens. These venues have been a pleasant surprise. We'd been expecting the kind of vast soulless sheds we'd played in 1990, the last time we were an opener, but these outdoor gigs have been smaller and much more conducive to music shows. There have been trees and spectacular views. I hear thunder but it's muted by distance, like a giant over the sea clearing his throat. Like somebody else's war.

We get the all-clear to start half an hour late, but people are still dribbling in as we play. Everyone enjoys themselves. Why not? It's play, after all. Who cares if I'm a bit old and rubbish? Who's embarrassed? I'm a spent farce. So what?

Catering is over by the time I've changed, so I happily go back to Mike's, which is miraculously open for another half hour. This time I try the vegan Philly Cheesesteak. Fuck me, it's good. I'm investing. I'm sold. If you told me there was a slaughterhouse feeding butchered cow carcasses into the back kitchen of this place, I'd believe it. I read up about them. Good local firm, food truck gigs and two restaurants. I want to get in on the ground floor. I'm going to make a killing, clean up, make a pile.

I watch the venue staff clearing up litter at midnight as the riggers and loaders dismantle and pack the production. These guys start early and finish late. You see them through the day, sitting in the shade around the stage looking shattered. There's a full moon hanging over them, bashful behind torn veils of cloud.

DAY 31, Nashville, TN

'Come on, baby.'

These words rouse me from a recurring dream. My Love can walk. This morning I knew she was lying to me. I wanted her to show me.

'Come on, baby.'

I pull the covers to my mouth, expecting tears. No tears, dammit. It's 9 a.m. and I take a pill and get out of there. Discouragingly, we're in a medical area, hemmed in by big hospital buildings. It's midtown Nashville and not too pretty: faceless multi-storey apartments, corporate hotels, all Sunday-morning quiet. I sit on a bus stop bench and a scrawny squirrel hops up to check if I'm holding. Nothing doing. I need coffee and a toilet, but I'm not going into a hotel. I navigate to the Well Coffeehouse where I queue with privileged young sorts, catching myself idly staring at the person's bottom in front of me. I am served by a girl so aggressively chirpy I fear she might be a malfunctioning robot. The coffee is a bit poor, but I'm grateful for the cool air within and warm chair without. There's an embossed iron historical plaque on a post a few yards from the patio celebrating Christian contemporary music, one of the hell genres along with nu-metal and classic pops.

I have my wide-brimmed cowboy hat from Portland today, which I'm mildly embarrassed by, but it's very practical in the high sun. No factor fifty needed. It has three holes on either side for cooling purposes. It's an entirely practical item although, because I am also wearing denim cut-off shorts, I think I'm more of a midnight cowboy. Wear it in Glasgow and the most likely response would be, 'Hoah,

Fannyman. Where's your horse?' For this reason, I intend to dispose of it before our flight leaves O'Hare. The looks of a twenty-something guy across from me reminds me I was dreaming about Lloyd Cole and the Commotions. In a toilet cubicle, I was telling Lloyd and Stephen from the group how much I enjoyed listening to *Rattlesnakes* the other day, something I did in reality. Of course, they were both their 26-year-old selves. It's how we see each other, we decrepit old musicians. We think we're still young and forget how ancient we look to everyone else. I catch myself lamely trying to pull rock poses on stage. It must be such a sad parody of what was once also sad parody but done with exuberance and elasticity. Because of the Ghastly Affliction, I can no longer move around while I'm playing bass, the difficulty in doing two things at once being one of the main symptoms. I have to kind of lurch between plucks. Dum... step... de-dum... step.

I keep dreaming I'm booked to do solo gigs and I have to excuse myself – 'I'm so sorry, I can't do this anymore.' The dreams don't worry me. The disease makes you feel too remote for that. You live in a kind of stupefied isolation behind invisible walls of numbness. All the time, the shadow inside is taking over, jerking your limbs like a puppet, making you vague, blunting what you hubristically thought was your personality. Where am I going? Where have I gone? Is everyone still here? I feel like I'm being remotely controlled by an unrecognisable version of myself.

Open-topped buses wheeze past, guiding tourists around Music Row and the rest of this unremarkable city's sights. I've never taken to Nashville. It feels like a cattle market for con artists. People sell song TITLES here; *I Wrote This Song to Make a Buck (Now Sing It, Fool and Get to Fuck)*. I prefer LA, as entertainment industry towns go. At least they don't profess to ownership of authenticity, that word that denotes the fraudulent. They know it's all fake. All the supposed history in Nashville is bunk. It's an artificial flavouring fortifying a bland brew.

Our old A&M Records fixer Al Marks picks Iain and me up for lunch. We sit in the swelter outside a health food place, munching salads. Al has to watch his diet because of his heart. He tells us his Vietnam stories again, always worth hearing. He has a mischievous bent tempered by a lifetime of surprises. There's a photographer at the venue who shoots us for a few hours before soundcheck. Allen is someone I've ended up knowing via email, so it was a risk to agree to let him shoot us, but he's super pro and we enjoy our time with him. For some reason, he insists I wear his Tom Ford specs. Not my type of item. But he's being playful, which is no bad thing.

Around six, I meet our friends from the '80s, Brigit and Kevin. Iain joins us on the porch of an adjacent coffee shop. They're wonderful, funny people from Little Rock – artistic and bright. We talk about death and dying, disease and depression, laughing a lot. There's not enough time. I check my watch and I am late for getting warmed up for the show. But we get to hang a little more in the parking lot at midnight after a few fans have drifted away. I don't mention the Ghastly Affliction to them. It tends to open up an avenue of conversation that's very one-sided. Al Marks has a photo taken with us backstage. He surmises it might be the last time, with his heart and our flagging career, and we can't contradict. This busy day has been a boon. I enjoy the show in Nashville's classic little rock club, Exit/In. A little rock, in Tennessee. See you in the next life.

DAY 32, Raleigh, NC

We changed buses last night, our original mothership's aircon melting in the heat. We're sad to see the old girl go, with her dark veneer and period wall lamps. The new bus, which I shall call the Strayhound, is a spiffy electric blue, her insides disappointingly dun. The toilet is on the port side and precious cupboard space is scarce, so there's the usual grumbling. Humans hate change. We just want to do the same things again and again but faster and faster. That's why this swap seems like a disaster. The Strayhound is like being on the old bus but after taking LSD. Everything's brighter and subtly altered in mysterious ways.

I do the day-off shuffle. Open case, put everything on charge and get out for a look-see. The hotel is located on an out-of-town interchange beside a large strip mall and one of those new zones that kids on it's a town, with the parking lot on the outside and square brick units facing one another through freshly planted trees across 'streets'. There are three pet stores. Where there's dogs, there's dollars. There are two supermarkets, a bunch of gym/health/beauty shops and a few chain food places. I opt for Cava, one of those make-your-own-salad-bowl joints – Subway for yoga types. It's hot like fire today. Seriously not walking weather. I'm irradiated in minutes, even with my cuntboy hat. What to do now? I lie on my bed and look at the car park. I tap some messages. Somebody. Help. Me. Please.

At nine, I walk back down to the mall, taking an outside table at a taco chain called Torchy's. I'm situated under a toppy JBL speaker playing pure pop. I've just been dozing to Irving Berlin, but now I'm staring down the barrel of Taylor Swift and Ed Sheeran's weirdly thin music. It ticks all the boxes that pop needs to tick – pretty tunes, catchy hooks, lyrics with a modicum of real feeling. It just feels like all the guts have been taken out. At the end, we'll be living underground, drinking the filtered urine of the rich while Elon Musk transmits this sonic anaesthetic from his throne on the moon.

DAY 33, Raleigh, NC

It's the 4th of July. The bus takes us the short hop to the amphitheatre. I step off just after noon. The heat is smashing from every surface. I see the surrounding skyline and walk out to find a city. The city is closed. The majority of the downtown infrastructure was not here last time we came through in the early '90s. A lot of high stuff got thrown up pre- and post-9/11. I find a grocery store, the clerk cashing up a guy who's complaining that, if he has no money, he can't get no girl. The store guy is about twenty-two, seems smart.

'Where you from?'

'Scotland,' I say.

'You goin' back?'

'Yes,' I say.

'You lucky.'

'I like it here. It's hot but it's friendly.'

'Some people,' he warns.

'Some people aren't so friendly in Scotland either,' I say.

It's a veiled conversation about racism and he smiles. But you can tell he's sick of getting shit from people.

I suppose you could say these cities of the South are maturing. Trees planted in the '80s now reach the fifth floor of the office blocks. Their populations are growing. But this heat gets worse and you worry about their viability. All around me, oil is burning, running automobiles, churning the aircon units. There's no silence in these towns. The chaos machine keeps gunning, pedal to the metal. The Stars and Stripes are out, fluttering in a flaming wind. A dog walker strolls by, the mutt's tongue hanging desperately from its jaws. A few homeless people weave about: a one-armed guy (a veteran or a junkie or both); a bench sleeper, her shoes on the sidewalk; a skinny meth wreck. Marvin Gaye's 'I Want

You' drifts from an outdoor speaker across the street. Birds shaded in the foliage chirp along.

I end the evening sitting behind the big outdoor stage as Barenaked Ladies ply their trade in the sweltering night. You can hear the fireworks. The surrounding buildings are lit up in red, white and blue. People have gathered on the roof of a multi-storey car park to watch the show for free, where the booze is cheaper and there are no rules. Let freedom reign.

DAY 34, Washington, DC

I'm up and running at midday in the positively bracing 32 degrees. I make for the National Museum of African American History and Culture, marching there at full speed despite the stew of swampy air and exhaust fumes. There's a palaver getting a ticket involving data entry on my device, a thing the Ghastly Affliction has made stressful. Gavin can be such a cunt on a phone. My index finger hovers dubiously before I point at a digit and the bastard often causes me to miss. Autocorrect is my saviour. And it's finally decided I use the word fuck a hell of a lot more than the word duck.

I tour round the museum starting, as instructed, in the basement and working my way up chronologically. It's very busy, but I look at a drawing of the chained bodies in a slave ship and switch off my moan meter. I hate to be flippant, but there's nothing very special about the museum itself, though the soundscape of washing waves in the early African slave trade section is affecting. And the maps and illustrations of pre-European exploitation Africa are enthralling. Some of the quotes, inscribed in impactful scale, are moving, but it leaves me unsatisfied. You glean much more from reading books, listening to records and watching documentaries. I don't find anything new or surprising here. I realise I don't like big 'important' museums. You feel as though you must absorb as much information as possible or you're a bad citizen. In an art gallery, you're the sole judge. If you hate it – stroll on. You're not in dereliction of duty if you sweep through a roomful of renowned abstract paintings you find ugly. You're just exercising arbitrary taste. You're free to be an idiot. So, I give the Holocaust Memorial Museum a miss. Because when does the coming together of profound historical subjects and mass tourism become a circus?

I take a riverside table at an overpriced oyster bar down at the marina by the venue. There's a super-yacht called *Neenah* moored nearby. The sky above is mottled with giant forests of cloud and jets appear above the tree line every minute. DC is somehow the most important city on Earth and the most irrelevant. It's a giant office dumped in a swamp. I think of David Foster Wallace's *The Pale King*, Alan Pakula's *All the President's Men*, Armando Iannucci's *In the Loop*. Bland, opaque and clerical. Square buildings, suits, square people.

After soundcheck, I wander along the marina promenade, one of those 21st-century developments: twelve-storey, high-ceilinged apartments, pedestrianised walkways, upmarket retail and eateries. There's a Gordon Ramsay Fish & Chips outlet and a Gordon Ramsay Hell's Kitchen restaurant. Another narcissist charlatan who likes to smear his name on edifices. I walk out on the only public pier I can find, the rest closed off for the super-yacht community. I sit on a swing bench, feeling the warm air slide past my skin. Behind me, the relentless roar of lifting jets thunders on. I hear a fake bell ring six times. An hour 'til showtime. I make my way back sluggishly through a throng of the wealthy.

It ends up being a proper rock show. Standing audience, loud room, great sound. Everything clicks. After we load out, I sit on a bench with Buddy on the avenue where the bus is parked. We watch people coming out of apartment buildings, summoning Ubers in the downtown heat. Dog walkers, diners, down and outs – the great hierarchy.

DAY 35, Red Bank, NJ

I get up late and walk around the neighbourhood of Red Bank. Gentrified for a long time, the quaint high street features stores selling collectibles and antiques and old cameras, and a music shop which is a kind of museum with vintage guitars and synths for four grand. I buy some plectrums. At 2 p.m., I meet Beth Tallman, our former promo woman and artist relations rep from A&M. She brings Emily, who was a radio plugger and whom I've not seen for years. We have a cheap Mexican lunch opposite the venue, which is a small club called The Vogel. We talk old people shit. Death of parents, retirement homes, aches and pains. Beth teaches music business studies to young aspirants. Beth is a no-nonsense, here's-what's-gonna-happen-type person. I don't tell them about the Ghastly Affliction. I don't think I've earned that concern. It's women like these, working our records in the States, who helped buy me a house.

I smile for selfies with fans after the gig, enjoying the beautiful New York/New Jersey accents. Maria wants us to pose with her giving me a kiss on the cheek again. I remember doing this last year. Why the fuck not? I walk to an empty bar in the warm blue night, take a seat and order a beer. A guy with tattooed muscles like bunches of bananas sticking out of his T-shirt shows the bartender pictures of his dog. He sounds like a goon from *The Sopranos*. I've never trusted sentimentality coming from tough guys. And I certainly don't trust their dogs.

DAY 36, Uncasville, CT

We're parked in the neon-lit bowels of a vast concrete complex hous-ing an arena, hotel, convention centre and casino. We're on tribal land again, this time the Mohegan, who traded along the nearby river now named the Thames. I glide up an escalator to what may or may not be the ground floor and break out of the nearest fire escape. I'm trapped in an empty yard, facing the wall of a parking garage. I find my way up to a road, get on a slipway and start marching down a six-lane high-way trying to get the fuck away from the prison of the venue. I have a coffee shop in my sights on the map. But I get picked up by tribal security. 'You can't walk on the highway, bud,' says Bill who offers to take me where I'm going. On hearing the word 'coffee', he takes me to a Dunkin' Donuts attached to a Shell gas station. He points out a sidewalk on the other side that will take me back to the compound. I tramp uphill to a massive, shade-less mall. No cafés, no trees, no benches. On the way back, I find a tiny local liquor store which has an extensive array of zero-alcohol beers. An Asian studenty guy comes in and buys four miniatures of Johnnie Walker. It's one of those places that's built onto a giant walk-in refrigerator behind the counter. I buy a six-pack of Becks and hike back. I find myself wandering through the complex in search of the venue. It could be an airport. I buy lunch in a food court below a skylight, which supplies the only source of daylight in the whole development. The decor is vaguely tribal and extremely well crafted, tiles and timber cut with precision and some originality. People are weaving about abstractedly as if they missed a flight out of here years ago and are stuck in a recurring nightmare of total redundancy.

I meander through the endless slot machines of the casino to the Bow & Arrow bar framed by a huge wall of screens showing every sport you might name. Zombified gamblers sit on leather swivel stools and gaze into lurid wonderlands of symbols and numbers, scrolling, scrolling, looking for the jackpot rush. Cleaning staff with blank expressions push carts around the fallen. It's the collective coma at capitalism's terminus. Halfway round this dimly lit circle of hell, I see signs to the Sun Patio where I join the lonely smokers and let the breeze lick away the smell of casino despair. Birds are chattering in the rafters of the bound-log, Native American-style structure supplying shade. A middle-aged woman dressed in white shares my picnic bench, smoking a kingsize and sipping a margarita. A band start soundchecking on a little tented stage. Entertainment, entertainment everywhere and not a thought to think.

On the way back to the arena, I find myself in a shopping centre. I start laughing. It's just mad. There's a Le Creuset outlet, a hiking shop, luxury handbags, jewellers flogging Rolexes and a series of indoor waterfalls, cascading over fake cliffs. There's an Irish pub (of course) and a nightclub. The waterfalls are so loud they drain out the piped pop emanating from somewhere in the roof. It's sensory overload from every direction.

We decide to do an acoustic set for the show as the arena is too ambient to handle complex frequencies. It works okay and a few of us wander back into Casinoland. Jim and Derek put cash into two hideous slots whose screens tower over their upholstered chairs. I watch their money go down, then up, then down, before drifting off to the roulette tables where I see two consecutive wheels hit zero and decide better. Not tonight, not here. A group of lovely east-coasters approach. They saw the show last night and have come up here to see us again. When they were all nineteen, *Change Everything* was the soundtrack to a formative road trip. We banter a bit and they leave me to my thoughts. The whole zone is a-throng with weekenders. The cacophony of it is overwhelming, like the sound you hear as you're about to die. The vast grim machine of it, hoovering in money and spitting out disappointment. I weave through the hotel foyer into the night. The air is thick with all the tears of slaughters past.

DAY 37, Gilford, NH

I have an indifferent sleep, having decided to forego the melatonin. I'm last up. I do my pathetic old man exercises in the back lounge for a few minutes and gather my things for a nosey. There is a flock of bone-rattler bicycles right outside the bus, which are free for us to use. I pedal, ungeared, down to the nearby lake, Winnipesaukee, but am unable to find access to the water's edge, private properties crowding the shore. But it's a pleasant enough ride along thickly wooded residential roads, a little black mailbox at the top of every drive.

Back at the compound, it's all very relaxed. The backstage area is expansive and kitted out with lots of outdoor furniture and pursuits – crazy golf, basketball hoop, table tennis. There's even a little games arcade. The outbuildings that serve the site are quaint wooden shacks. Our dressing room has its own porch, mature forest all around. It has a holiday camp vibe. François, our talented French-Canadian monitor engineer, breezes by on one of the bikes. Single-engine aeroplanes drone up from the nearby airstrip. I watch Carlos, our merch man, throw a few hoops. He looks pretty decent to me but what do I know? The first thing we noticed coming to the States in 1986 was how well-developed all the guys were. They had upper body muscles you never used to see in the UK, all their high school sports being hand sports. But nobody could kick a ball for toffee. The thought of throwing a ball makes Gavin quake with fear. I can't throw for shit anymore. Christ, some days I can't write.

The Bank of New Hampshire Pavilion really looks after its artists and crew. There's a kiosk beside the campfire set-up backstage dispensing cocktails and, at end of play, a food truck appears serving tacos and hot filled rolls. I nurse one of my non-alcoholic Becks at a table while idly trying to smash fat mosquitoes in handclaps. I'm in my bunk early and watch the Apple TV Velvet Underground documentary. I once had lunch with *Interview* magazine contributor Danny Fields, invited by A&M press people, not knowing what a legendary part of the '60s avant-garde and '70s punk scenes he was in New York. I told him I recognised his name from a photo credit on the reverse of Steve Forbert's first album cover, which he found wryly amusing. I'm suddenly reminded how futuristic the Velvets were with the first album line-up. It's easy to forget what a unique and beautiful racket they made, blending instrumentation in a way never heard before or since. Drone pop. God, I love them all over again.

I fall asleep to a Barbara Stanwyck film, having long, complicated dreams about people I know in incongruous settings. I wake at seven and peer out at a gloomy Boston harbour. Everybody's asleep, the Atlantic laps in, suggesting the madness of civil war.

DAY 38, Boston, MA

I meet Fred Mollin, Jimmy Webb's producer, for lunch in a big seafood restaurant right next to the Leader Bank Pavilion. These New England banks do like naming sheds after themselves. Fred looks as fit as last time I saw him nearly ten years ago. He listens to my troubles and tells me stories about legendary '60s songwriters. I feel like I'm pouring my pain into him, but Fred's a producer; he feels it, empathises and says this: 'Justin. You and me. One fucking record.' I can't argue. He gives me six CDs – his recent productions – and I rattle them in the back lounge disc player when I get back. People from my band say: 'Why so perfectly middle of the road?' Don't they know, right time right place, me and Fred are going to tear the world apart? Fred once offered me a fully budgeted album, recorded in Nashville, remaking Billie Holiday's *Lady in Satin*. I said no. That could have been the biggest mistake of my life. But I'm holding out for a future project me and Canadian/ Jewish/Europhile Fred can do. He's never made an ugly record. I want to persuade him to start with me. Fred, it's the ugliness that makes music perfect. This man got me singing with Lamont Dozier. That overdub alone opened up an area of Black music to me hitherto undiscovered. Fred is a friend. He's America. He has ears like a lynx.

As I walk back through the venue, I see a crowd of people onstage, realising that all the bands and crew are posing for a group photo. Perhaps I missed the memo. Iain recommends the ICA and I go looking for some culture.

I pay my twenty bucks and squash my bag into a locker, choosing number four. Four is for the Beatles and the original Del Amitri line-up. The perfect number for a small ensemble. A combo, a group. With five, it becomes a band. I start on the top floor, enjoying the sculptures by Simone Leigh of eyeless – and sometimes faceless – African-looking women in ceramic. Two figures have spoons for heads. One figure's whole head is a hole, rimmed with raffia roses. There are vaginal clam-shell heads, huge grass skirts and an abstract mound edged with braided rope like enormous sutures from a clitoridectomy. The next room features lovely work by María Berrío, big paintings rendered in Japanese paper painted in watercolours. The pictures feature haunted children. One, called *Cavalry*, shows two young boys on a carousel, a man with an iPhone snapping from a secluded distance appearing almost indecipherably in the centre. The gallery leads to a glass-walled corridor looking onto the harbour, busy with the wakes of a hundred pleasure craft. I walk back along a pristine boardwalk, passing two yuppie walkers with those pot-ugly hounds that seem so popular. In-bred, snuffling lumps of ill-fitting flesh on mutant skeletons, wheezing on their leads like survivors of some terrible experiment.

The show is a bit of a struggle. I take my third pill of the day right before the gig. The fuckers don't really bed in for an hour, so I got that wrong. I worry unduly about my pitching, miss a lyric and get stuck on the bass a few times. The Ghastly Affliction is exasperating. Things run smoothly for a few hours or a few days and it suddenly appears to remind you of your impairment. It's like a mental illness in a lot of ways – you're doing battle with yourself. You try to control it using reason and logic. You try to trick it away, but it floats like a menace ready to strike at the oddest of times. It plays utter havoc with your confidence and, as we all know, performing is a game of confidence. The voices spinning in my head onstage – hit the note, remember what's coming next, don't get ahead of the beat – mix with terror of what the disease might throw at me. It's impossible to relax. And you put every flaw down to its effects, when some of the inaccuracies (lack of vocal control, a missed beat) could conceivably be a result of age or tiredness. It's one more big doubt keeping you from being the performer you know you can be. But I'm happy to be here and hear people clapping.

Andy has an accident during the Barenakeds' set, tripping on a cunningly concealed metal bar and hitting his mouth on an aircon unit. I see him go by in a wheelchair (!), the medical people looking thrilled to have something to do. He looks like he might need stitches on his upper lip. God knows where they're taking him, but tour manager Mr. Fudge is in hot pursuit. Messages from the emergency room keep us updated on the WhatsApp group. Andy seems upbeat, but it's an anxious wait to hear how he gets on.

Derek has the bus drive down to the hospital as the waiting room is getting scary. He's relieved to get out of there. After a few hours, Andy emerges with a thick lip, four stitches and a prescription for blood pressure medication. It turns out he lost all his pills when he left his toilet bag somewhere and didn't bother trying to replace them. I don't think it explains the stumble – his blood pressure was high not low, so it wasn't like he took a dizzy turn on standing. I checked the place where he tripped and it looked almost designed to fuck you up. We eventually haul out of a deserted Boston around 3 a.m., glad to be whole again, feeling good to be moving.

DAY 39, outside Buffalo, NY

The bus is parked by the hotel very much in the middle of nowhere. In fact, I soon ascertain we're on the periphery of nowhere. But there's an all-day breakfast place fifty yards away, so I order a Californian crêpe and coffee to kill time while waiting for my room. Derek pops in and puts my key on the table. The waitress says, 'Now you have somewhere to stay'.

'It would appear so,' I say.

I'm not up for walking – the map shows nothing of interest. I take a few hours to trawl through the entire Barenaked Ladies catalogue. Jesus, there's a lot of it – albums every year or two from the early '90s. I unearth a couple of jewels and gain a better understanding of what they're trying to do. They've endured one major change of personnel, the founding member and principal singer and writer Steven Page drifting out of focus around the turn of the tens. The records steadily improve from then on, proving the exception to the rule that bands who continue beyond the departure of their lead singer are always an inferior version. But in BNL's case, most of the early songs were co-written with Ed Robertson, so there is more continuity. But it's not really my cup of tea, this stuff. Too cheery and clever. But some of it is funny and some of it quite touching. And, boy, have they worked hard. And meeting them and being so kindly treated makes it impossible to be too scathing in any analysis.

I walk to a rotten Mexican at the next mall along the highway. This is the worst of anywhere on tour, hiking for food under trash-strewn flyovers, over endless parking lots, gargling fumes. I'm in a mild strop. Later, I watch the Australian film, *The Stranger*, with an exceptional performance by the UK's Sean Harris. In spite of its threatening mood and macabre theme, it cheers me up. It's pleasurable to find something unexpected of such good quality.

DAY 40, Lewiston, NY

I spend the short ride to the venue in my bunk, dozing and listening to music – Link Wray and Shilpa Ray. I decide Wray's 'Fallin' Rain' might make an excellent cover until I discover that cool bastard Father John Misty has recorded it. Fuck.

Andy is sitting in catering at the venue looking most displeased. He's obviously in a lot of discomfort and needs his blood pressure medication badly. There's some confusion about what is being done about this, but a bag of pills turns up after the soundcheck courtesy of a runner. This was immediately after I'd handed him a blister of my beta blockers and he'd taken double the dose I'd told him to take. I don't think he's thinking straight and is probably mildly concussed. He cheers up later on, but it can't be fun being stuck on a bus with a badly swollen lip and teeth moving about.

Before the early show at six, I hike along the Niagara River gorge on a path that winds round cliffs a few hundred feet above the fast-flowing turquoise water. The other side is Canada; I see the maple leaf flying by a hydroelectric power station on the opposite bank. I meet Louis, Iain's son, sitting on a rock halfway along. He has an unlit joint in his hand, rolled with brown papers. Maybe he forgot a lighter. I talk to him later after the show and he seems quite baked. On the hike, I spot an orange bird, the colour of fire, flitting through the trees. And black butterflies with wingtips of orange. Louis had seen a chipmunk. Stick that in your iSpy book.

The Artpark Amphitheatre is small with a grassy hill far off to stage right that looks like a slide. It is redolent of a village fete. I feel very much as if I'm phoning the performance in. I try to kick myself up a gear but it's not easy finding the impetus to play to a few hundred mildly interested spectators in the late afternoon. One's mind wanders. I worry about Andy. I think about home. The absolute heartbreak of it. Yesterday, as I sat outside the awful Mexican restaurant, I gazed at the unedifying view and thought, *my life is fucked*. As the end approaches, I feel myself slipping back into despair. My angel disabled, my mother gone, my time running out. I keep reminding myself to be grateful for the present. But I never liked the present; it was the future that excited me. So I wall myself off and live in the small cylinder of the now. It's warm, there are people, there's a river.

DAY 41, New York City, NY

This could be the last time, baby the last time, I don't know.

I love New York. Did I nearly move here in the '90s? Was I going to get engaged to Susan, the smart, sneering New Yorker? I don't think I had the balls. Fantasy. I'm a craven little home-boy. Since the big gentrification, the planes, the colonisation of Brooklyn, New York has slowly got back its mojo. The pandemic has helped – a lot of the rich have simply not returned. It won't be long before J.J. Hunsecker can say again, 'I love this dirty town'.

New York isn't America. The Velvet Underground, Grandmaster Flash, Robert Mapplethorpe, James Baldwin, Debbie Harry, the Ramones, Television, Patti Smith, Allen Ginsberg, Jackson Pollock, Thelonius Monk, the Actors Studio, the Yeah Yeah Yeahs, Patrick Bateman, Patrick Melrose, Paul Auster, John Dos Passos – they're not American, they're New York.

Pier 17 is way downtown on the East River, so I dogleg north, stopping in a few little squares I find on side streets to collect my thoughts. Everyone has attitude – the suits, the hard hats, the teeming masses. They exude a stoic pride and brazen confidence. They wear looks of earned exhaustion. Even the pigeons have a sassy strut. Everything is alive, the city throbs with the meat of life. It's an engine that runs on human blood. There are characters on every block, the stick-thin old queen with dyed hair, hipster girls in headphones and mini-skirts, the service guys with tool belts, the Central American couple arm in arm going for lunch, he in construction duds, she in a summer dress.

I walk up Broadway a few blocks and angle through Chinatown and Little Italy, crossing Canal at some point. I pass a guy with a handwritten sign, citing an episode of police brutality. A fat guy is ushering him from his pitch. The fat guy uses the N word among other shit. The other shit is wildly racist. I'm talking slaver vernacular. Slaver vernacular – on the streets of 2020s New York. I tell the racist guy to shut up and ask the protester if he is okay, but he's oblivious. He walks off pretty pronto. I follow him down the cross street on the opposite side. He doesn't need me, he doesn't need white defence. He needs people to read his sign.

I get to east Soho and start looking for a fuel stop. I'm in need of a restroom so dive into a bar that does all-day brunch. Isn't brunch always all-day? I order a breakfast burrito and the barmaid asks if I want any protein on it. I say no. Does that mean I have foregone the eggs part of breakfast? I have no idea. The restroom affords little privacy for my ablutions – a sink and a stall behind a thin curtain. I notice Gavin has been quiet today – this city is so distracting. As I sit, I feel his hesitant frailty make itself known. But I'm happy. I'm sitting in a tree-lined street in NoLita in the heat of the New York summer, birds twittering, the traffic muted.

Recently I've become concerned with what people think of me, what they're saying about me. This is a new thing. I never cared before. I wonder if it's paranoia caused by the affliction when it occurs to me that the longer you live, the more complicated a memory you leave behind. Failures and successes, happiness and ill health. You die at thirty-two and you leave a clean legacy. At ninety, half of it is pretty bleak. Your changing opinions, your encroaching irascibility. It gets complicated. I don't wish to be remembered for being unwell. These are the things that drive the vain to suicide. The desire to be dead invades your thoughts. But cowards like me don't have the heart to bring it down. Besides, I don't want to be a drama queen or, like Holden Caulfield, leave a bloody mess.

I meander back south. I sit and watch handball players thumping rubber balls off a concrete wall between Hester and Grand. Two guys are excellent, punching shots with impressive pace. The courts sit in the mottled shade, hungry sparrows flit about my bench. Predictably, the right-handed athleticism causes Gavin to shake in envy. There's every kind of people around here: young mothers with prams, old coots in baseball hats and braces, meditators, derelicts, a film crew. There's a handsome guy shuffling around the handball court trying to bum a light for the half cigarette that's been hanging from his lips for an hour. Everyone is blanking him. A regular loon, I imagine.

Four guys get together for a doubles match. I've seen Andy Murray play tennis and this is better.

Near the venue, I go into an Irish pub for air conditioning and a bottle of Heineken 0.0. They're playing Blondie's 'Heart of Glass'. There are four men in the whole place, spaced three stools apart along the bar, tapping at their phones in a vignette of male loneliness. As I walk down the street from the pub, I hear a voice calling my name beguilingly. I turn and realise it is fan not friend and pose for a two-shot. The woman has the loveliest broad Long Island accent. I warn her of the early start, smile a goofy smile and flounce off.

The venue is on the rooftop of a new warehouse-style development with commanding views of Brooklyn and Manhattan, the Empire State peeping out through a crack in the skyline, Lady Liberty off to the south. Six black helicopters fly overhead following the path of the East River. I have a small epiphany while we're playing 'Driving With the Brakes On'. The sun is lowering behind the towers around Wall Street and lighting the frontage of Brooklyn Heights like a Canaletto. Planes are glinting as they come in to land and I'm singing this song for the thousandth time. It feels like a fitting farewell to this city I have loved so much since I was twenty-one. I have this magical image in my mind, those high buildings standing sentry in the Atlantic currents, as I call into the wind with the Brooklyn Bridge behind. I sing through their gates. Everybody at my back is the West – the free world.

I have dinner with our manager, Andy P, and two of his old friends. It's a brief glimpse of a whole other world – Reuben is an architect and Julie is in sustainable fashion. They have kids at college and an apartment in Brooklyn. They caught one of the new ferry lines to be here. I don't imagine they thought much of the show. I struggle to muster my social self. I'm perilously close to ordering a drink in the loud, over-lit and overpriced restaurant, but I manage to steel it out.

Andy Alston with his bloody wound comes by and takes a seat and a glass of rosé. We talk about Prince Harry, colonialism and a failed unpoliced drug project in Philadelphia. I run back up to the rooftop, where the Barenakeds are finishing up, to find a journalist called Stuart with whom I've been loosely corresponding. With his girlfriend, the three of us make a fast exit down the escalators to a margarita bar set up on the side street right by the tour bus, waiting like Cinderella's coach. The reassurance of the warm night air holds me in its dark embrace, the talk is engrossing, the cool drink goes down like a sleeping draught. Why would you ever leave this town?

DAY 42, Wilmington, NC

Rain is teeming down, my hotel window a blurred square. I lie abed in my black boots listening to it lash the thick glass. I'm behind the waterfall. I look at the sad little plastic amenities sitting in a line on the dresser – coffee maker, ice bucket, TV. I have no mission yet, no restaurant or gallery to go to. I lie in limbo.

The storm clears at three and I am navigated to a Mexican fifteen minutes away. It looks confusing inside. It has a sandwich counter and I don't know why this should be. There's a sushi gaff next door and the rum characters that greet me there are sufficiently odd that I take a seat outside in the muggy afternoon. A branch on a nearby tree cracks and severs, thudding on the asphalt. That rainstorm must have been the last straw. Waterlogged.

The gap-toothed waiter has the air of someone who's either served time or served his country. He utters too many 'sirs' and calls me 'bud' with a sinister lilt. Turkey vultures circle overhead. We've seen a lot of those on this trip. One hovered over the stage at the Niagara River while Andy was missing from the soundcheck the day after his accident. I thought, *Oh, don't say he's pegged it*. He materialised shortly thereafter. He wasn't having a good day, the endorphins having worn off overnight.

I hole up in my third-floor room, falling into a light sleep listening to music. A song by Courtney Marie Andrews nags me awake around nine and I fiddle with the map, thinking about dinner. I'm not hungry but might be later and all the places within walking distance are closing. It'll have to be the wings shop. I take the plunge and sprint across the six-lane highway that forms the major physical barrier between me and food. It's pitch dark and I stumble a little, but it cuts out a ten-minute detour to access the nearest crosslight. Buffalo Wild Wings is a cavernous shed with scores of TV screens strung high around the walls. I can see ten different sports from my booth. For inexplicable reasons this awful place cheers me up. It's the first time today I've felt part of the town.

I'd been reading Wilmington's Wikipedia page, and front and centre is the Wilmington insurrection of 1898, also known as the massacre. Once a thriving Black-majority town, the largest city in North Carolina, Wilmington was an exemplar of racial integration with African-Americans holding significant economic and political power. But a conspiracy of Democrat white supremacists put paid to all that, staging a coup d'état and using a non-existent 'race riot' as a pretext to expel Black citizens from political office and destroy Black-owned businesses, eventually leading to a reduction in the African-American vote from 125,000 to just 6,000 in six years. It's only in recent times that these grotesque tragedies have been brought into the light of mainstream history. The same shit is still happening with voter suppression, a racist criminal justice system and a lunatic far-right Supreme Court. In capitalist systems, it seems, someone is always being punished, someone always has to pay.

I eat my repulsive bean burger with my wayward hands as the staff sweep about my feet. The big lights go on. I know when I'm not wanted. I make the mad dash across the black highway to the hotel. I hear frogs and crickets sing in the sultry night. This land is their land.

There are eight shows left and I sense the looming melancholy. What will I do with nothing to do?

DAY 43, Wilmington, NC

I dash to the bus in another downpour and, on parking up near the venue, I wait for a break before I head out to explore downtown. It's a steam room out there. I find the high street in minutes and buy some novelty socks and an umbrella in Cape Fear Footwear. It's Jim's birthday today and I find a pair of socks emblazoned with the phrase 'More Cowbell'. I still regret not buying a pair in Amsterdam that depicted a hippie guitarist plugged into an Orange amp that read, 'I AM the band'. To this day, I have no clue why I didn't buy them for Iain. Blame the hesitancy that comes with the Ghastly Affliction. Blame it on the GA, blame it on the hippy-hippy-shake, the boogie, the night, put the blame on Mame. If you've never seen *Gilda*, do. I decide this is what my songs need – melodrama. Some days I think they need radical simplification. They need something. I order coffee and a smoothie in a chic little café. Kale, spinach – you know the deal, you metrosexual cunt. I'm on North Front Street facing beautiful brick turn-of-the-century facades. Which of these housed Black-owned businesses before the purge?

The heat of the sun ricochets up from the white concrete sidewalk, the wind like a hairdryer. Two blonde beehived ladies cross the street in floral pantsuits and matching gold-rimmed sunglasses. They look like extras from a B-52s video. I imagine that they imagine they are Southern belles. The smug white pedestrians look like they know what they did, these still-victorious ethnic cleansers. The ghosts of nineteenth-century freedmen haunt the street; you can picture the crowds in their finery. What a scourge white folk are, what a pitiless plague. A bunch in branded T's from some convention offer me bottled water from a little cart they're dragging. 'Sir, would you like a water?' I shake my head in silence as I slurp my green sludge. What are they, the Christian Rehydration Squad? The clouds close over and the fat drops begin bouncing off my table. I shelter inside and watch the wind shake the saplings.

Everywhere you go – art gallery, coffee shop, tattoo parlour, truck stop, deli or shoe store – they're selling T-shirts and baseball caps with logos. The world is awash with these wasteful souvenirs. We sell this sort of shit every night, clogging up the future. The human race will end up fashioning entire cities from these cotton and polyester remnants. Shanty towns will be named after obscure lube shops, kids will cower under Del Amitri blankets on their MAGA hat mattresses.

I walk down to the Cape Fear River where slaves were traded until fewer than 160 years ago. Wilmington is a port city, sited inland on a deep navigable waterway. The battleship USS *North Carolina* is moored on the far side, a WWII fighter sitting on its deck despite it not being a carrier. I think about the extraordinary tonnage of sunk shipping in the 1940s, the extravagant waste of it all. I take a look into the Museum of the Bizarre, but it's too sad and too busy. The sun is beating down, stirring the sludge of the air. As I head back to the gig, I see a giant cloud bank of gunship grey, like a wall of doom. I up my pace and try to beat the rain.

It stays dry for the show and afterwards I eat a little, toast drummer Jim's birthday and head out into the still-blue evening, walking along the river towards town on a newly built promenade, past house-boats and yachts. I sit at a bench facing the water drinking in the humidity and tranquillity. Couples amble by, and there are still a few solo dog walkers abroad. I can hear crickets and the sound of the water gently lapping against the boats. A band is playing somewhere, a female voice carrying on the heavy air. I have entertained and now I'm done. I wish the warmth would swallow me up and spit me into eternity.

DAY 44, not near Valdosta, GA

Bad sleep, bad dreams, but I pill up and am out in the swamp heat by noon. Iain tells me there's a zoo, so I go looking. Backstage is a dis-mal shanty town of tumbledown huts and loose gravel. The trucks are doing a coordinated shuffle and stirring up dust. The woods around look like jungle. This is south Georgia, practically Florida. There's only one bog for about forty band and crew, so I use the theme park facil-ities on the way to see the animals. The zoo is spread throughout the theme park. You find yourself staring at some endangered species of marsupial while screaming kids fly overhead, hanging from mad con-traptions. First up are two squeaky-clean squirrel monkeys – basically squirrels with brains and prehensile tails. Gorgeous things you could sit on your hand. 'Roll to Me' strikes up from a tinny speaker and I move away.

Two three-toed sloths lie still as rocks in a cage, one with a forepaw hooked on a branch, so immobile it's like a sculpture. Opposite is a pair of snoozing raccoons looking dejected, like over-medicated patients in an asylum. One casts its glance in my direction as if begging for a mercy killing. Next-door, ring-tailed lemurs pace about haughtily, their long tails swaying straight up. The males have black scrotums like olives. I've never even heard of a coatimundi before, let alone seen one.

Squat badger-type things with sandy coats, they sniff at the ground with slightly upturned noses as if disgusted by the smell left by a recent guest. They are currently putting up with horribly jolly fiddle music coming from the alligator enclosure.

The fennec fox with its yellow fur is about a quarter of the size of its European cousin with huge hyper-alert ears. The fake cactus in its shed looks like a comedy prop. The fallow deer are all asleep in their paddock, probably glad to be unpopular, but it can't be fun living next door to the alligator show. The macaws are as big as rugby balls and look down on me with avidity. The green monkeys aren't green and have been spoilt with a big fake waterfall. On a tight turn, I get stuck in a pram jam before the black bear habitat. I struggle to spot them when a massive pile of fur raises a long arm, looking strangely simian. This guy has a sweet territory like an English country garden.

An albino garter snake pink-eyes me from behind a dirty pane, weaving its head in a figure of eight motion as if to say, 'You're not all that, human'. Wandering back, a squirrel shoots across the path and fires through a hole in a fence. Why does *she* get to be free? An enormous porcupine sleeps under shade, like a witch's broom with a face. Black dragonflies zip about. A lone turtle floats in a puddle like a lost mariner. Two wild boars lie camouflaged in wet mud as if victims of trench warfare.

The wooden walkway winds around a swamp forest of water oak and red cypress, passing a cage of beautiful diamond doves, tiny and delicately speckled, like hand-painted porcelain. They have big red buttons for eyes, their heartbreaking call mournful and pleading. I'm struck by a wave of grief, so I savour it, imagining my mother here, saying something funny. I sit on a bench on a deck that faces the swamped forest, with its green carpet of tiny plants on the water's surface, the thin trunks rising elegantly from flared bases 80 feet into the sky. I hear screams from a rollercoaster somewhere. The sun hammers down on the untamed wilderness in front of me, the denatured hellscape of the theme park behind.

I find myself alone with a caged African grey parrot and make pathetic throaty noises I'm guessing might be its native tongue. She regards me with disdain, refusing to play ball. Don't all parrots parrot? I journey onwards, the burrowing parrot not burrowing, the laughing kookaburra stern-faced. I imagine there's not a lot to laugh at when imprisoned behind four walls of wire. Beyond the swamp, I nose into Tiger Tales where a trainer is having a young cat show its chops. I catch the finale where the tiger climbs up a fence to snatch a morsel from its keeper's stick. I'm longing for a mauling.

Our show is a thirty-minute set in front of mostly bored holidaymakers. We come as close to phoning it in as we dare. Catering – which is the sort of hut with open sides and insect screens you might see in an outback-set Australian movie about toxic masculinity and racism – is closed. I walk out of the arena, which is just a big car park with a shed at one end, and find the nearest amusement park fast-food stall, enjoying a thoroughly repulsive pulled pork sandwich. The stuff I squirt on it to disguise the foul stench is made out of kerosene. I wander round a few more exhibits. A spider monkey is making unspeakable gestures at a prairie dog in the next cage. His little pink penis looks like a raw Wall's sausage. The poor creatures have to suffer all-day marimba music coming from those stupid outdoor speakers that are half-buried in the ground like huge sprinklers. They must be stressed to breaking point and must long for the night, to fear the day when all this hell shall start again.

DAY 45, St Augustine, FL

I'm last off the mothership after a long sleep accompanied by Eric Hobsbawm's *The Age of Revolution*. The heat is thuddingly wet, and the map shows little within a mile, so I break my habit and have lunch in catering. At lunchtime. This is the life of the crew – stuck all day at the venue, never seeing anything, not even the immediate environs of the site, always at the end of a radio. I put on some laundry to make use of time. Our dressing room is spacious and has a wall of mirrors with make-up lights like a dressing room should.

I sling my smalls in the dryer and take a quick look around after a heavy downpour. The cute bijou amphitheatre is surrounded by a thick jungle of pines, palms and shrubs. I meet a security guy who directs me to a pond.

'Just go down to the dock, there's a turtle there. Make some noise and he'll come right to you. There's a dock.'

'A duck?'

'A turtle.'

Several turtles surface to peer up at me standing on the dock. I count two big, three little, all with algae growing on their shells. The pond smells pretty ripe. Thunder bellows in the distance. I imagine this is a perfect day for turtles, gloomy with spots of rain. They're awkward swimmers – going down seems to take a lot of effort. The water is alive with little fish which might be tadpoles, I can't tell in the green murk. The rain has a welcome cooling effect. After the early show and food, Andy, Iain and I are driven to the beach by CK, the amphitheatre manager. CK is telling us how their venue beat Red Rocks this year for the National Outdoor Arena Award. He says a lot of other stuff, but I can't hear him over the noise of the golf buggy engine. We walk through loosely vegetated dunes to a long, deserted strip of coarse white sand.

The waves plunge into a trench before flattening on the shallow shore, dragging the sand from under your feet on the backwash. Iain has a long swim, Andy a dip, I a paddle. I lie flat on the sand and bend my neck back to see the sun setting behind me. I feed some gulls crisps from a goodie bag furnished by the venue. About thirty come squawking around, effortlessly catching morsels mid-air. Two black-headed gulls arrive trying to intimidate the smaller birds, so I make sure they get nothing. When the bag is done, I stand and flap my arms to shoo them all away. They fly up like a pleasant surprise.

We are three old men on the beach, dithering about. How terribly odd we must look.

DAY 46, Charleston, SC

Finally in a Carolina that isn't North, tonight is the last of our six headline shows. I've been asleep for twelve hours and am scuffing up King Street by midday, walking north until the retail runs out and turning back. It's the standard gentrified shit – women's boutiques full of linen dresses, coffee shops and vitamin bars set in charming nineteenth-century Main Street-type facades. I have eggs with corned beef hash and grits in Toast! across the road from the Music Farm. I ponder how all US food is (with rare exceptions) the same: very prompt and served with cheese. I manage to avoid the addition of cheese to my grits at the last moment. Prompt because it's all about profit and cheese because it's cheap and adds fat and salt. The diner has bad music. But it's forgiven for the big, clean and private restroom – two square metres of personal space – a luxury after a long night on the bus. I cannot wait to get a few days of privacy. Without alcohol to ameliorate, the entourage gets suffocating. You begin to resent people you love. You begin to resent yourself.

I walk south on King Street, past endless upmarket gifteries, T-shirteries, scented candleries, and one shop called Yeti that just sells thermos flasks and coolers – for suckers. There's a decent record shop, but I've got all the records I need. I'll use Tidal if I want some hi-fi. In a bookshop, I read the first page of *Will*, Will Self's memoir. It reads well and I make a note to pick it up at home; I have enough weight. I turn left towards the river and see what appears at first to be an anomalous office block, as if a bit of 1980s Berlin has been dropped onto this genteel jewel of the South. A cruise ship! All is explained. These horrid little bric-a-brac outlets are the honey traps set for the herds of grazing cruisers, brain-dead and stir-crazy after too much lobster and too many mojitos. Cruise ship cunts! Bleed your dollars into this parasite town! I take a side street route back to the bus and get caught in the rain. I shelter on a fake marble memorial bench under a broad tree in a churchyard. Some panicking cruisers stumble about the roots, as if the rain is poison. I pass Pounce, a cat café. I peer through the tinted glass. A young black and white is luxuriating in the caresses of a twelve-year-old boy. $15 an hour, says the sign. Fully booked 'til three, says another. Ten minutes would do me. I'd talk sense to the twelve-year-old for four and get the motherfucking moggie on my lap for six. Job done.

It's one of those long, slow soundchecks. We start early and Iain is too far away to join for the first hour. The four of us rehearse a song called 'Sometimes I Just Have to Say Your Name', which we want to try at the Bandstand in Glasgow. I find the lyrics grating – very sentimental and a bit of a lame attempt to be the Faces – but it gets a lot of requests because we never play it. Probably because it's shit. But we are nothing if not servants to our audience. Simpering and pandering, we must appal so many other groups as so many appal us.

I have an early dinner in an awful Tex-Mex restaurant. Sitting outside, as I always do, I get selfied twice. The standard pose in these situations is to stand in the middle of the group with your arms spread loosely around the others' middle backs in a pathetically feeble impersonation of intimacy. I worry that meandering Gavin, trembling as he often is, might one day be misunderstood.

I walk east through a poor but smart neighbourhood to find the river. Brackish waves lap at a patch of yellow sand and I take a bench to gaze out past a moored paddle steamer to a sleek deep sea-green aircraft carrier, echoing Wilmington. I count six fighters on deck. Low on the waterline with well-hidden gun ports, this thing looks way more scary than its World War II ancestor on Cape Fear. I'm pretty sure it could waste me, and everything around me within a hundred yards, in a second.

Later, I have a rest on a bench opposite the County Library. A couple, around my age, are dragging all their worldly goods behind them, their cases piled high with bed rolls and sleeping mats. They seem like they're looking for shelter. They probably had a house a few years back. Now they're internal migrants, refugees of a system that doesn't want them. I look at my suntanned wrists, the hair there going grey. First I've noticed that. I'm snowing over. I walk a little further and see the couple have joined other itinerants in a small park, hidden from view from the street. Back on King Street, I'm arrested by a sax player across the road. I lean against a palm trunk and listen. Beautiful tone and delicate phrasing, with his baseball cap and shades – I perceive him to be a serious old dude, but when I cross to put five bucks in his cup, I see he's nineteen. I want to invite him to play a solo at the show but I'm too shy.

It's not much of a turnout, maybe a hundred or more people in a big room that could squeeze 600. It's one of the ugliest-sounding rooms we've heard – horrible high mid-frequencies bouncing off the arched ceiling and brick walls – and we all struggle to find a way in to the show. I'm grimacing at the squealing noise I can hear in every chord, but the crowd stick with us and appear to enjoy themselves. I sit on the bus with the band after, nursing a Heineken 0.0, regarding the smokers hanging outside a late bar with mild envy. But I'll be glad to be gone. Up to Virginia and the last three gigs in the big tent.

DAY 47, Portsmouth, VA

I organise – pill, water, pass, nicotine patch, hat – and make for an art gallery, the map leading me to a route across the Elizabeth River. I pay four dollars for a return trip on a quaint paddle ferry. Everywhere I look are warships – cruisers, destroyers, battleships, a high carrier wrapped in white plastic to keep spying eyes away from top-secret repairs.

It's hot and the twenty-minute walk around the edge of down-town Norfolk is not pleasant, but the Chrysler Museum of Art is. Free admission and a locker for my satchel. This large building, designed in a renaissance style in the 1930s, now mainly houses the Walter P. Chrysler Jr collection, a vast heap of treasures from antiquity to the present spread through fifty airy rooms. I start on the ground floor in the extensive glassware area, some funky Italian objects from the 1950s making me smile. In the ancient world section, the Pre-Colombian stuff is great, with a couple of ceramic deformed infants and a life-size warrior whose armour was reputedly made from flayed human skin. I read this, on the wall:

'After the Maya gods created the world, they made humans to do their work. The first people, fashioned from clay, crumbled when they tried to speak, and the second group, made of wood, spoke mindless chatter, so the gods destroyed them. When the gods made humans from corn, the people spoke wisely and were gifted unlimited vision, much like the gods themselves. Worried that people were too powerful, the gods weakened human sight and their vast understanding. Now amazed by the universe, the people worshipped the gods and set out to explore the world's mystery.'

There's a stunning Frank Lloyd-Wright window and incredibly delicate cosmetic vessels from impossibly distant eras. I gaze at three exquisite Egyptian heads. It's all looted, stolen with dollars and the power they bring. Upstairs, the only painting that really stops me is *White Factory* by Niles Spencer from 1928, a flat, perfectly proportioned cityscape from, it says here, the Precisionist movement. It's the closest thing to a masterpiece in here, the Gauguins and Matisses being some of the worst examples of the artists' oeuvres. Old Walter Junior had the cash, but I don't think he had the taste. There's an instantly recognisable James Baldwin, in mustard and lemon yellows by Beauford Delaney, looking a little teary in 1965. And I like Henri Laurens' *The Bather* sculpture and a lovely *Head of Balzac* by Rodin, fist-sized and staggeringly modern for 1880. Three hours fly by and I step back into the heat thoroughly satisfied with my visit. The ferry back is cool and delightful.

It's a friendly crowd, but as usual we play to a slowly filling empty house. We can see the masts of four ships from the stage, poking over the ridge of the usual lawn at the back of the amphitheatre, this one largely covered with one of those stretched marquee-type roofs of white glass-fibre fabric. It sounds good. Post-gig, I walk up to the local drag and nurse a zero beer outside a run-of-the-mill neighbourhood bar. You don't get the feeling anything very exciting ever happened here. It's a student crowd and the slightly cold bar staff are playing Michael Jackson. The church bell across the street tolls nine dull beats and I remember I'm due my last pill. The Cinderella curse again.

The pill sharpens me a little and I'm alert and bored. I watch the last third of the Barenakeds, still utterly bemused to be watching my bandmates on the big screens during the 'supergroup' finale. I wrack my brains to come up with a way I might contribute on the last night – something funny, something good – but I'm out of inspiration. Things have gotten so awful in my life recently that I don't seem to care any more. The problem with all of this is it's necessarily a mediocre facsimile of an energy-fuelled 1990s – for the players and the audience. These 'hits' being played are more than thirty years old. It's sad and it's tawdry. We're end-of-the-pier entertainment driven on by dribs and drabs of money, milking it, one last turn around the block. Of course, it's not what I wanted to be. I wanted to be an 'artist', probably. But I'm a veteran cretin. I should be gotten rid of. I should be history.

Around midnight, I wander out onto the venue concourse. Staff are shutting up concession stands, a man is pushing plastic dumpsters across the tarmac. I sit by a marina looking across the river to the navy yard and that wrapped-up warship I'd sailed past earlier. A tug glides quietly past. The night is old and the raison d'être for everything is draining away.

DAY 48, Philadelphia, PA

For your cheesesteaks, I don't care, Philly, but I love your narrow streets and grubby grandeur. I head south from The Met, the refurbished opera house on the seamy north side, through non-distinct, hard-to-figure neighbourhoods, to mill about town. Every museum and gallery is closed on Wednesdays, so I'm aimless, without mission. I've been warned by those in the know that Philadelphia has some dodgy areas at the moment, a Christiana-style open drug market scheme going badly wrong. Town is as pleasant as I always find it – busy, friendly, brisk. I don't come upon much to look at and it takes me a while to find a place for lunch that's local and suitably mid-market.

Last night I had terrible, apocalyptic dreams. In a country house in the Scottish Highlands, all hell broke loose, the mountainside beyond French windows opening up into a volcano, spewing ominous grey filth into the sky, chips of ash and stone tapping at the glass. Behind the mountain were cooling towers also belching thick columns of black smoke. The radio was reporting a meltdown in Latvia. I shut the windows and filled the bath.

I'm in a foul mood, I realise. An awful, staccato call from home with my very ill angel. Muggy air, nowhere to go. And a day off to come, five miles outside of Akron, OH. I was hoping there might be a Devo museum, but we'll be lucky if we're near a shop. I usually feel a sweet pang of melancholy at the end of a long tour, but I hate the band on after us so much I don't want to take part anymore. I detest them and am having trouble being polite to the singer. Perfectly nice chap, you understand, but you'd need to be super charming to surmount that shallow, sentimental shit he slings every night. Aahh. That's better. I inform Kris and Andy that I've decided to take a drink. They don't demur. I think I've done pretty well, eschewing alcohol for three months.

After the show, I dash out to meet friends from 1986, Jason and Pat, and we have good Italian food in the old Lorraine Hotel down the block from the Met. We talk music, music, music and a bit about ageing and infirmity. Pat's a bit older than me and Jason, who was a young lad when I first met him. Pat has run a record shop all his life and Jason has been writing about music (and, more recently, sport) his whole career. So the three of us have, somehow, bizarrely made a living for forty years from the thing we love. We walk back up to the venue as the punters stream out at the end of the Bares. I get selfied a few times, but the faint warming effect of two beers with dinner make it less awkward than usual. I'm back on the bus at midnight and, for me, mayhem ensues.

DAY 49 AND 50, day off, outside Akron, OH

The first thing I remember is finding the hotel bar around closing time. I order a beer and get talking to the staff. Michael is behind the jump, Bruce and John take stools and I buy them all a drink. They don't stay long and regard me quizzically. Who is this intoxicated Scotsman? Bruce, I'm surprised to hear, wants to go to agricultural college. He looks hipper than that. John is young and shy, Michael a happily settled gay man who has vague ambitions to move state. I pay up and get back on the empty bus making a few calls home, thankfully not getting through. You have to get through to someone. At some point in the night, an enormous electrical storm passes through, frighteningly heavy rain shaking the bus, lightning popping a few metres away. This storm, we hear later, caused the cancellation of the show the night before ours, 21,000 people held under the amphitheatre roof until it was deemed safe they could leave.

Thankfully a few of my colleagues come aboard after going bowling, an excursion I drunkenly slept through. Carlos the merch man commandeers Iain's speaker and we sing Beatles' songs and he plays Del Amitri's 'I'm So Scared of Dying' about four times in a row. We accept the compliment. After the bus empties of both alcohol and bodies, I take a notion to look at my hotel room for the first time. I enter, turn around and go straight back to the bus and get into my bunk to begin the recovery process. I lie in suspended animation for ten hours, surfacing around 3 p.m. to mope around what I can safely assume will be a ghastly soundcheck followed by a 'challenging' show. I don't disguise my condition to anyone – what would be the point?

The thing is... I don't drink any more on the road. Looking after the voice and all that. But sometimes a wave comes speeding in from the ocean, from a hundred miles out to sea, saying drink me. Drink me. I take the plunge. Oh, the sea is beautiful.

The show is hell, of course. I need more breaths for every line and find it extraordinarily difficult to hit any notes square on. My bass playing is all over the shop. I feel regret and pity for the few fans in the auditorium who paid to see this. They seem weirdly enthusiastic. I feel very similar to the time in 1990 when we played Tipitina's in New Orleans after we'd all taken acid on the day off the night before. The sound of our music clattering around the walls is vast and monstrous. Everything seems over-amplified – the sound, the colours, my nerves. I'm straight back in my bunk after dinner, Eric Hobsbawm's *The Age of Empire* audiobook nursing me into a dream-rich slumber. My girl is well again and walking in a weird world. We go out for dinner in a strange foreign city. As I open a taxi door for her, I notice my hand start to shake. Reality makes its unwanted entrance. You can only push the snooze button so long. At some point you must wake up.

DAY 51, Pine Knob, MI

I'm up at noon, hugely dehydrated but well slept. We played Pine Knob Music Theater in 1990 with Melissa Etheridge, but I don't recognise any of it. I hike off site to a mini-mall at a nearby intersection and get cheap Mexican food in a chain. The waitress is solicitous and regards me with wry amusement. I load up on carbs and Coke, the American way. It's been cooler here, up north, 23 degrees feeling chilly by comparison to the absurd heat of the South. It's good walking weather, but I can't see anything worth walking to. Besides, there's a bloody great golf course around the venue limiting routes out. Golf – the parcelling-off of open land for the exclusive use of the rich and hateful. I'd ban it. Jolly reggae is piping from the ceiling of the restaurant and I take my leave.

I walk around the venue – the usual covered auditorium with an open lawn at the back. It doesn't sound quite as cavernous as last night. I have no idea what my voice will be up to this evening, the last show. It could quite possibly be worse. I dread the soundcheck. But physically I'm better. Oddly, I was so hungover yesterday that Gavin didn't have the energy to shake. But he's back with a vengeance today, wobbling away at my side like a little engine. O, little yellow pill, do your work, give me strength, give me perk.

The show is good. I think: *I can do this!* I can't, of course – I have Parkinson's. I cannot do much of anything. I cannot whisk eggs. Or, I can but no longer with the elliptical motion I had perfected over decades. Sometimes I just move the fork violently in a stuttering side-to-side frenzy like a scratch card addict who's reached bottom. I cannot walk downhill or downstairs without applying conscious determination. I noticed this on my first post-lockdown hill walk. I fled up to the summit in great enthusiastic leaps, but on the descent, I felt as though I was suddenly too tall, my feet too far away, my body a top-heavy structure about to topple. Other recently liberated walkers streamed past around me, my pace stupidly slowed by a sudden sense of vulnerability. I put it down to lockdown lethargy at the time, but looking back it was a sign. Maybe deep down I recognised the difference. I didn't feel unfit. I felt feeble and infirm. I felt like I shouldn't be on that steep path down a mountainside. I've not been on a hill since. There's enough going downhill in my life to be going on with.

I attempt to get pissed in the dressing room after the gig with my friends Bobby and Mike, but it takes me a while to get into the swing. There's a champagne reception with the BNL lot on a patio somewhere, but I'm told it's only for the touring party, so I stick with my guests.

We drive the five hours to O'Hare, those of us still drinking horsing the last booze on the bus. There's just about enough. The big old mothership pulls delicately into the hotel car park like a submarine nosing into Atlantis. I sit up front to watch the ballet of CJ manoeuvring the enormous vehicle right up to reception. Goodbye battleship, you protected us well.

The plane will lift, as planes do. Take me back to my angel, take me back to that glue.

DAY 52, O'Hare Airport, IL

Today's interest mainly involves Andy losing his passport. Derek has made arrangements for him to stay another day at the airport hotel so that he can go into Chicago proper tomorrow, when the UK embassy will be open and able to issue him temporary documents. It's not been a lucky tour for Mr A. He thinks he probably lost his documents on his way to the dentist after his accident. So, there are only four of us flying to Glasgow with all the gear.

I'm on the plane, I have not lost my passport. But Andy was my roommate for years and years so a brother to me. Before I leave, I say to him: 'You lucky bastard – you get two days off in Chicago.' Chicago. The one town in the whole continent that, via two big radio stations, made me and Andy feel like we belonged. Del Amitri all day long. Made us the most-loved small stars in a very big town. Andy – it's Chicago. He cheers up.

On the journey home, buckled into my window seat, I don't look out. I don't take measure. I stare at the small screen in front of my face, watching endless entertainment. I'm coming home to a broken boy, only son of his mother – herself destroyed by life and those of us who live it – back to a son, a woman and a planet I temporarily no longer understand, undermined as it is, every day, by not being America.

I arrive, fall into bed, fall out again. My stricken baby smooths my hair down, calls me Owl. Owl. I've been nothing of the sort. I've watched and left to let her suffer. I cover her with my wings and she whispers: Where have you been?

MIDDLE EIGHT

I live a double life.

On the road, I have a routine, I'm occupied. At home, I do little. I find it hard to get out of bed, as though I believe if I stay very still, no other calamity can befall me. I cringe in the corner of the empty kingsize and peer into the glow of other people's lives on a laptop. For days at a time, my whole world is on my lap, flickering like a fucked puppet show.

I venture out – the odd movie, a night of debauch in the pub carried on at a flat – and weave home under cover of the pre-dawn deserted streets to begin the repair of my disrepair. The cycle starts again. Each day I cringe with guilt and remorse until I force myself to get in gear and get on my bike to visit my care-homed broken Love. I chain the frame to a fence around the little garden her room looks on to and walk around to the main door to be buzzed in. I'm visiting a jail exclusively populated by the falsely convicted. The staff are, without fail, sunny of disposition and sympathetic. I knock and enter My Love's room, as if checking on a bandmate in some economy hotel. Sometimes she's abed, sometimes sitting in her wheelchair waiting, endlessly waiting. I'll kiss her awake or whisper her name. We'll sit and gossip and I'll read her the news from my phone. She will interject with memories obliquely jogged by random words and phrases. And because I know her so well, I can locate each story from her past with some gentle inquiry. It's not always easy but sometimes we laugh a lot. We will sing a bit. I'll help her eat. Occasionally she'll admit that she loves me and my whole world goes on fire.

In November, I manage to cajole myself into making plans. I book the borrowing of a house from my friends' often-absent neighbours in a remote hamlet on Lewis in the Outer Hebrides. It's a hideaway I've taken advantage of many times before – an island off an island off the mainland island, the perfect place to write. I get fourteen songs done in six days. I have no idea if any are much good. I'm just glad they're out of me. Let that stuff live in the tape machine, not swimming round my breast. It's the first batch I've written since the whole pile-up of last Christmas and there's not much daylight in any of them. But if a song wants to exist, who am I to deny it? I just let the poison flow and am done with it.

I'm strapped for time, so only manage a couple of short walks around the ragged coastline. I watch the sea smash distant cliffs like white fireworks. I survey the silver Atlantic, turquoise fringed in shallow bays. The whips of winter air fill my lungs with the wilderness. It's medicine.

On my last night, I smoke a congratulatory cigarette and say farewell to the sea, looking out to a lighthouse and the cold expanse of ocean beyond. Sheep shuffle about in the gloom. I catch an early ferry from Stornoway and take to the deck to watch the ship's slow easing into the embrace of the Ullapool hills. It's one of the most beautiful harbours in the world. I gun my little black car through the dark glens to my city in the south. I have a haul of trophies in a tan briefcase in the back. Pleased with myself, I shall now return to the routine – binge, hide, work.

PART TWO

DAY 53, Aberdeen, UK
1 March 2024

I'm in a first-class train carriage at Queen Street Station in Glasgow, waiting to depart for Aberdeen. Today I am no man of the people. A long-haired lawyer called John is rabbiting on, excusing his new hirsute image as a result of lockdown. Fifteen years ago, he represented me in 'a traffic matter'. I vaguely remember him. We had briefly convened in a side room at Perth Sheriff Court to confirm my guilty plea to a string of speeding offences. This was the era of peak speed camera. The fuckers were everywhere, lurking round sharp bends in country lanes, crouching in bushes, mounted on the far side of overpasses. I happily accepted a six-month ban, hardly missing having a car at all. I even got papped on the way into court, the accompanying *Daily Record* headline reading, SPEED KING. That same quick black car, bought brand-new with ill-gotten cash from dodgy dealings in the early zeros, dropped dead two days ago, the clutch disintegrating beneath my foot. I knew immediately it was terminal. After more than twenty years' faithful duty, the scrapyard finally beckoned. I handed over the paperwork to the nice lady in the garage who arranged the funeral. Another totem of my virility consigned to the past. Farewell speed king.

As I gaze through the carriage window, the late winter light mines gold from the gleaming landscape, from the yellowed grass in the pastures to the tiniest of buds pushing through on bony-fingered tree branches. I'm set to daydream my way north when John the lawyer reappears for a gossip. In my experience, criminal lawyers are extraordinarily voluble. If you listen carefully, all sorts of vital and fascinating information streaks through the stream of conversation, like veins of fat in good red meat. We discuss Celtic, our team, and bond over mutual disdain for sectarianism. The old hatred still blooms in its various hotbeds, rooted in anti-Irish sentiment from the nineteenth century when Irish migrants flocked to Glasgow to escape rural poverty and took poorly paid jobs in heavy industry. The hangover from this ancient prejudice still consumes us in Scotland. It seems to me that vestiges of this nonsense will survive as long as kids are sent to separate faith-based schools. At the same time, I can see why a Catholic minority would want to maintain its cultural identity through various institutions. But, in my soul, I'm a secularist and want gods nowhere near education. I want them nowhere near me. If gods exist, they're weirdly coy. If they're omnipotent, they're profoundly sadistic. And if they purport to love us, why are they so twisted? Gods are gangsters, lording it at the top of the food chain, ordering hits and mutilations in sanitised code, keeping their hands clean.

Tonight, I appear with a roster of other singers to perform the songs of Burt Bacharach. I have found my allocated tunes hard to learn and almost impossible to inject any feeling into. Hal David's lyrics are mostly plot with the slightest peppering of poetry and serve the rhythm and the melody far more than the reverse, indecently subservient to the demands of Burt's cleverness and complexity. Burt's world is one where the clothes do the walking, the person a puppet of their immaculately tailored power.

I'm not confident about the evening. Gavin has been restless in rehearsals and I am getting distracted by his fluttering about my face when trying to hold the mic. And my voice, if I'm honest with myself, feels fragile. The train pulls out of Dundee, the sun glinting on the wide mouth of the River Tay, the sky a pale beseeching blue. The light, slashing in from an angle, is startlingly vivid. At this time of year in Scotland, the whole day is the golden hour. I feel my body relax as Glasgow recedes. The nagging domestic drudgery, My Love trapped in her body, spoon-fed like an abandoned lamb, bills, repairs, admin. The Ghastly Affliction has impaired my ability to cope with simple things like emails, form filling or travel arrangements. The slightest snag sends me into a panic. I deal very badly with minor crises. It's like I'm suddenly eighty-five and lost. I am lost. I have lost. All this losing – people I love, skills I had – is an undressing, a slow dismantling. I look out of the window; a meadow slides by. At its centre, a hare lies dead as if victim of a parachute failure, its winter coat ruffled by the breeze.

I'm sitting on a sofa on a stage, squinting through the spotlight beams. Ross Wilson of Blue Rose Code is performing a few feet from my black patent shoes. The audience are silhouettes just beyond the event horizon of the apron. The other singers sit around me, egging on the current turn, waiting for their cue. I have a moment of deep contentment. It's such an uncommon sensation I take note of it. I'm ecstatic to be onstage in the middle of an event, surrounded by a little orchestra of delight – flugelhorn, clarinet, piano and string bass off to my left, brushes and vibraphone behind. At my right ear, a string quartet swells and shivers in sudden patches like a caress. This would be heaven for a blind person – a 360-degree sonic experience. The winter has been hard; this is suddenly all so easy.

And yet it isn't. Compared to the Barenaked Ladies' shows last year, surrounded and anchored by my band – my bass at my waist serving as a shield – I feel terribly exposed. I'm alone at the front with just a microphone. I make unusual mistakes. I get a cue wrong and get up to sing when it's not my turn. I haven't managed to memorise the lyrics after a month of practice. I'm flummoxed when one of my song sheets slips from my music stand. I fail to look comfortable onstage. I'm off my turf, out of my zone, struck dumb in the spotlight. Del Amitri has been a harbour and a kind of hideout from the Ghastly Affliction.

I've been singing many of those songs for thirty years and they're burned into my memory like childhood. I can conceal my symptoms within that familiar world. I always know what's coming next, so I can devote my energy into battling the disease.

But in this milieu, singing somebody else's tunes with a band I've just met, I have to be alert and I just don't cut it. Situations like this demand an extra jolt of adrenaline, but adrenaline, once so vital on high-pressure shows, is now my enemy. It massively exacerbates the tremor and confusion. I can tamp it down with beta blockers, but then lose any edge I have left. So, when the slightest thing goes wrong, here I simply flounder and freeze up. I have to admit that I'm probably beyond doing anything outside the security of the Dels. A group is a gang and gangs protect their members. I hadn't realised how much I'd come to depend on them. With Iain, Kris, Andy and Jim at my side, backing me up, I feel like I have a fighting chance. Without them, I'm just an old fool, incapable of leading from the front. Where once I felt like I could be the point man on any stage, I now feel myself leaning back into the line, taking succour from their support. It's both tragic to me and enormously reassuring. Like finding out that love, after all, can keep me alive.

And, of course, all the time the Affliction chips away. Every few months another simple thing becomes stupidly difficult. Tying my shoelaces, putting on my jacket. Cuff links are no longer a viable option. I dread buying new clothes, imagining the laughable wrestling that may ensue in the fitting room. What were once avenues are now obstacles, opportunities now impossible hurdles. The way ahead is strewn with indiscernible roadblocks; simple actions once so automatic are now a challenge to be met with strategic thought. I faithfully pop my pills and wait for the little lift, but with each passing month, they lift a little lower.

After an early breakfast in Aberdeen among the tight faces of com-mercial travellers, I loll about in bed all morning, deciding to take a later train. This gaff's bathroom mirror is softly lit and exceedingly kind, so I don't experience the usual horror of the full-frontal decrepi-tude. Everything is still blotchy and crumpled, but not the complete flash-lit crime scene I've come to expect. This affords a good start to the day. My train flows south under a surprisingly high sun. Spring is coiling tighter just around the corner. I pass through Montrose, see tiny fishing boats beached on mud. The glittering sea sweeps out to the left, fields and copses to the right. The soil is rich. Last year, climate chaos wiped out a vast percentage of the potato crop up here. The tubers swelled, rotted and washed away in the constant deluge. I see golfers, all of whom I regard as twats, pulling their little wagons of implements about like deluded prospectors, looking for the rainbow's end. Two filthy horses stand in a paddock in tartan blankets waiting for riders. An army of clouds approaches like a mountain range on the march in gunship grey and tattered white. The muscle of the engine is hauling me home. Home is where the hopelessness is.

DAY 54, Glasgow, UK

I lead the house, room by room, into darkness, leaving a note for My Love's son Luke, who is to cat-sit. The taxi looms out of the rain at 10.30 p.m. and ferries me to the bus parked up in a post-industrial hellscape on the Clyde. The rain makes rivers in the gutters. I heave myself aboard and am gratified to discover the same bus we hired for our European tour in 2022. My name is on my usual bunk. Lovely Simon is the driver. Nothing has changed.

We are overnighting to Leeds to join Simple Minds on an arena tour. I have been looking forward to this. I have enormous respect for the Minds and was a fan of their third album, *Empires and Dance*, as a schoolboy. They brought a shiny modernity to dismal early '80s Glasgow. They adopted a Cold War European vibe in contrast to the subversive jangle of the Postcard groups. You could dance to Simple Minds. They united the geeky post-punks with the hairdresser crowd, driven by their automated grooves and noirish scenarios.

There's a bug going around. Iain sounds dreadful – like Daffy Duck. I feel pretty rubbish and have been so for a few weeks. Will the sting of the stage blow this virus away? There is the usual air of excitement at the start of a tour – the chitchat is bright and swings between nostalgia and practical stuff. I fear for the general mood should this virus take a firm grip on us all. Derek gives me two capsules of paracetamol for good luck. We stop for fuel south of Glasgow and I take the opportunity to sniff around the chocolate selection in the garage shop. Two police officers are buying coffee. I immediately think I'm behaving like a shoplifter. I summon up that half smile of acknowledgement as they pass me on the way out, a smile that tries to communicate respect but betrays fear and contempt. I probably look like I'm holding in a fart. I skulk back and undress for bed.

I remember this bunk. It's all crazy angles and crisscross stitching. When you read for a while then quickly look up, it all slides around your visual field like an acid trip. It's most disconcerting. The movement of the vehicle on the tarmac is gentle and comforting. I'm in a cradle. I have been craving this cradling.

DAY 55, Leeds, UK

I pop a Parky pill at ten and go downstairs. Kris is sitting in the front lounge looking a bit stunned, but says he slept well, unusually. I tell him about the book deal and he asks how I feel about being 'outed' – a radio doc and TV interview about me and my disease having recently been broadcast. It does feel odd. I stepped outside my front door a few days ago and a builder accosted me.

'You're the man from the telly!'

'I don't know what you mean.'

'You're retiring...'

What, precisely, I was supposed to say to that was lost on me and I mounted my bike and left him in the lane like a lost dog.

Kris says I seem a lot better than before, but I'm not sure which 'before' he's referring to. But that sentence alone gives me a colossal boost. All the afflicted want to know is – am I normal? Am I weird? I'm thankful that I live in an age when disease is no longer shameful or seen as divine punishment. But there's much embarrassment about it. People don't like shaking – it makes us uncomfortable. It's perhaps an evolved trait. Keep away from the trembling man, you might catch it. I suppose you could claim that every kind of cruelty and viciousness is an evolved trait. Murder, torture, rape – the law of natural selection says these behaviours must have conferred a survival advantage. But, of course, that's a just-so story. Animals display all sorts of ludicrously wasteful behaviour. Evolution never perfects. It blindly hammers out freaks and chimeras.

The bus is tucked under the towering Leeds First Direct Arena. Banks are so keen to get their name paired with entertainment. They hate to be perceived as just boring banks. Banks want to be nightclubs. The last time I went into a bank, I thought I'd mistakenly entered a spa. They've spent so much effort trying to be consumer-friendly, they're now being replaced on the high street by the very businesses they've been impersonating. Now you can't talk to a teller; you can only bank on there being a barista. I grab my tour pass and head for an art gallery. I might as well continue where I left off in the States, drifting aimlessly through public institutions by day, quaking in my bunk at night. Leeds is warm and windy. Ripped low cloud scrapes across the steeples. I sit in the big window of a coffee chain and admire the facades. The contents of my fruit cup and coffee have been flown in from far-flung outposts of the old empire. Imperialism's not dead, it's just disguising itself as democracy, that magical essence the West insists on spreading about the planet as a panacea. It's the same old exploitation. Extract resources, pacify the natives with Jesus, divide and rule. Instead of Jesus, they now preach a soft-power Hollywood version of liberty. You are free to be used by the wealthy as long as you vote correctly. If you don't, we sponsor a war.

I talk to a couple from Northumberland who are in town for the show. They ask me how I'm keeping and I can't decide if it's a loaded question. They're very sweet. I hear about a wonky hip replacement and the outsiders who've flocked to their town since the Covid catastrophe. They have glowing skin burnished by clean country air.

This is the odd thing about having gone public with my Parky. In the States, six months ago, only my US friends knew and even some of them I didn't tell, not wishing to burden the conversation with anything heavy. But now the audience are aware, it's been a curious experience. Fans have been so kind and so earnest in their sympathy. I feel it incumbent upon me to appear light-hearted and insouciant. I don't want to bore them and I don't want to get too personal. Fans aren't friends, no matter how supportive. Both parties want to keep a certain distance. The tricky thing about being unwell is that it's impossible for people to express their concern without that distance closing a little. It's hard to negotiate. Some folk try to be humorous about it and can get it a bit wrong. I feel for them. What do you say? Overall, it's been a huge relief, not having to hide Gavin's giveaways. And it's been a revelation sensing the genuine love people have for the work we have done. Maybe the slight shortening of that no man's land, between performer and audience, has been the one positive facet of all this rotten unravelling.

I tour round the art gallery, the usual municipal hodgepodge of tatty contemporary installations and nineteenth-century oils. There's the Tiled Hall Café to the left as you enter, looking like a great bazaar. I briefly admire Antony Gormley's *Brick Man* model – never built but stunning. It's much more impressive than the *Angel of the North*. People were to have entered via the figure's heels, to climb inside and peek out of the eyes. There's not a huge amount to see as refurbishment is under way. I could do with some refurbishment myself. I enjoy a large portrait of a 'Lady in Black' (who is 'Entranced') by Hubert von Herkomer. She gazes out beyond her frame like a nonchalant visionary. She's a poser par excellence. There's a nice little depiction of a Melita from 1931 by Ronald Ossory Dunlop. Her hair is torn like thick wool. I sit outside in the plaza, watching two drunks take turns on a plastic bottle of cider. A Henry Moore sculpture, *Reclining Woman*, lounges on her plinth above them. She could be equally sauced.

I wander off to the retail district, doglegging through the famous arcades. I pass Dame Vivienne Westwood's outlet – another fraudulent rebel who went ga-ga for a gong. Show me an English iconoclast in their twenties and see the simpering toady in their sixties. I take a seat in one of the larger arcades, beautifully restored and gleaming with some decent modern stained glass in the lofty apex. The flat vowels of the Yorkshire accent catch my ear. 'No' is pronounced 'Neh'. After so many months marooned in Scotland, it's exotic.

I go back to the bus to find Iain languishing downstairs with a lost voice. Uh-oh. Daffy Duck has turned into Tom Waits. There's been some laryngitis going about. Singers live in fear of such things. I'm now frightened. And I've been feeling unwell for weeks now. I cross my heart and hope not to die.

I peel back out to the arcades. In an underwear shop, the till girl calls me 'sweet' as she hands me my receipt. It lifts my spirits for an instant. The city is swarming with empty high-end boutiques. Some of the old arcades are exquisitely tiled and decorated. I keep treading on.

Back at the venue, I watch the Minds do their soundcheck party. They play three songs and take questions from a group of a few hundred fans with gold passes. They do a note-perfect version of 'I Travel' – one of the great hits of Scottish rock music. Jim Kerr is very charming and relaxed. I think these people are getting their money's worth. Jim comes into our dressing room for a chat before our show. He's wry and well-seasoned, and I find his charisma irresistible. Part of me is the teenager in thrall to his band at Glasgow City Hall in 1980, part of me honoured to be treated as an equal.

Our set has a few first-night hiccoughs, but it's the best I've felt all day. After a grim few weeks, I'm thrilled to get through a show in one piece. We watch the first half-hour of the Minds from the wings and are impressed. It's art rock on an epic scale and tailor-made for big rooms like this 8,000-seater. I go out front to hear the mix, but am waylaid by selfie seekers. Some just want to shake my hand. They seem genuinely pleased to meet me. This is the trouble with big screens. Everyone recognises you when you go front of house. I decide to take a walk in the cool evening air. Things in town are surprisingly tame for ten on a Friday night. The pubs are quiet and the chicken shops empty. Maybe this city kicks off a little later. In Glasgow, by now nobody walks a straight line. As I head up the hill back to the bus, I watch a man in a wheelchair propel himself along a bike lane, pausing periodically to take a bite from the sandwich in his lap. I somehow have the feeling he would not be amenable to the offer of a push.

DAY 56, Manchester, UK

I pass two security checkpoints to get off site, finding myself under a series of three railway bridges, sharp shafts of light angling down between them. The sky has lifted and Manchester is domed with the most beautiful blue. I navigate to Evelyn's, the first place that comes up when I punch in 'breakfast'. This town has effected some of the most courageous urban renewal in Europe. At every turn you meet mad collisions of the industrial past and the near-present. Glass boxes grow out of old sandstone ramparts, nineteenth-century red-brick facades cage 21st-century offices. Concrete car parks jam up against Victorian terraces, old warehouses, sunken canals. It's bewildering in its energy. Not all of it works, but the sum of all this building on, and referring to, the past is intoxicating. The music I grew up with has much to do with this renaissance. From Buzzcocks through Joy Division and Factory Records to the Smiths (not to mention those towering outsiders the Fall), bands made the new Manchester. Music played a crucial part in establishing the creative cauldron of this dazzling city, sucking in designers, artists, writers. Put a pin in the place and pivot the country upside down. London is still looking down on Manchester, Scotland is still looking up.

In Evelyn's, the morning hubbub is building, Saturday is starting, the Bee Gees are trilling 'Tragedy' and babies are crying. It's essential on arena tours to get out for breakfast, lest you find yourself permanently encamped in the daylight-free environs of some concrete fortress. It helps if the weather is good. You can roam more widely, sit on public benches, people-watch. The wind and rain drive you into the sad clutches of retail interiors and your mood dips accordingly.

As I follow my nose around the low-rise streets of the Northern Quarter, I find myself inevitably retracing my steps of three years ago.

The geezer in the Afflecks vintage clothing stall remembers me. I bought a brown three-piece suit which I've never worn. Lapels on the waistcoat – that's the problem. I get stressed buying clothes. I don't want any fuck near me, making little comments, judging me with a sideways glance. As I am trying on various jackets in the cramped space, an American couple come in. I just know the lady is going to comment. She will not be able to help herself. When I try on a smart long wool coat, she mutters, 'Nice fit'. I turn immediately and, as politely as I can, warn: 'Never interfere with a gentleman when he's shopping for clothes.'

Thankfully, she smiles. I buy the coat. The shop owner tells me about doing a job he hated in Glasgow, fitting cigarette gantries. I'm momentarily confused – he means those plastic display cases you used to see behind the counter in every newsagent. Now fags hide in secret drawers like treasure in safety deposit boxes. Hidden fruit. I sit on a wooden bench in a small square at the back of the football museum, a visitor attraction that has never attracted. Two girls in loud Saturday outfits sit at my back in a storm of perfumes. Manchester City fans flow past – they play Newcastle later. Qatar versus Saudi. Across the square sits Chetham's School of Music with its turrets and gothic windows like a haunted country house from a Daphne du Maurier short story. It's just about warm enough to bask for a bit, if you keep your limbs tight to your body. I arrange to meet Sal and Diane, two fans from 1990. We can't believe we've not seen each other for six years. Touring in a Covid bubble caused that. I feel spots of rain and turn tail for the venue. Two pigeons, fat from fast food, flap away inches from my head.

Tonight's dressing room is another windowless enclosure, a breeze-block holding cell. It has two vomit-coloured leather sofas and an entire changing room of cubicles. Large LED-framed make-up mirrors face one another on opposite walls, creating an infinity of receding mes. It's a corridor into hell. Kris has been pondering infinity recently, seeming to suggest that an infinite universe makes everything meaningless and non-existent. It's a bit above my head. I joke that the mirrors reflecting one another do not create an infinite number of reflections but, once reduced to a certain size, reveal a tiny Jimmy Savile. Speculation stopped at sordid.

After the show, I discover we are sailing to Ireland in the morning. I was dimly aware there were shows in Dublin and Belfast, but had no idea they were so near the start of the tour. I quite like all this living in the moment. Everything is a surprise. If only life at home could be thus. But recently it's been a daily diet of sadness and distress. Waking up each day to remember My Love is in an institution a stone's throw across the Clyde from our house is a constant disaster. See my friends, way across the river.

DAY 57, Dublin, Ireland

I come to suddenly in the blackout of my bunk and feel the telltale sway. I have missed the roll-on and must remain onboard the bus in the bowels of the ship for the crossing. I'm blind – I have no internet access, so can only glean the progress of the voyage from the swell below. I sense we are mid-passage. From a window, I dimly make out John McConnell Racing emblazoned on the side of a horse carrier. It has seven little portholes, but I see no horses' heads. Still, it's firm evidence I'm on the right ferry. Dammit. I love crossing water and watching the land recede to the aft and reappear to the fore. I love gazing into the turquoise wake, the great churned V reaching out in yearning to what's been left behind. I feel like Matt Damon on Mars, abandoned by my crew, alone on the mothership in the belly of another. I decide to put some clothes on, make the best of it. I may be alone, but no need to let things slide. Must keep the spirits up. I hear a muted cough. Somebody else alive! I am saved!

The cougher is Jim, who also missed the chance to get off the bus. I sip coffee in the downstairs lounge, Jim telling stories about his experience recording with Simple Minds in the '90s. Their writing/recording process would be best described as experimental, working songs up from riffs and grooves, looping and editing. It's the opposite of the lone troubadour strumming in her garret producing a complete song – top-line melody, lyric and chord sequence nailed down before it leaves the room, the only variables left to fuck with being key and tempo. With the experimental approach, everything is up for grabs. Ideas can start in one place and end up in another entirely unrecognisable one. It leads to much more original destinations. It's how we used to work in the early '80s. We'd plug in and I'd say: *Who's got an idea today?* Someone would play a figure on a guitar and we'd all work out what to add to it, effectively playing in a loop for ten minutes. Then we'd start the process again. Eventually, we'd find bits that could be joined up with other bits and I'd write out an A–B–A–B–C type structure and we'd record that sequence. Those bits of paper might read like this:

CHRISTMAS BIT × 2

C JANGLE × 8

BEEFHEART BIT × 4

CHRISTMAS BIT × 2

C JANGLE × 10

F JAM × 8

BEEFHEART BIT × 8

I'd take the cassette home at night and write lyrics and melody over that semi-organised piece of music and, the following day, we'd tweak it, re-record it and start all over again. We did that every day for two years and wrote twelve songs. It was hugely labour-intensive, but the few songs we produced could only have been written by those four people in that room. No single person could have come up with such mad contraptions. That's why our first album holds a unique place in a few people's hearts.

The rest of the gang suddenly pile onboard, ruddy with St Paddy's Day morning pints of Guinness. I absorb the rosy bonhomie jealously. Within a few minutes' drive of the docks, we're at our hotel, a newly built glass-and-steel shitbox – airport-style and echoing like the halls of hell. You take an exterior elevator to reception, then an interior one to your floor. My room is a big shoebox with the en suite wedged at an angle in the corner. It takes me three minutes to work out how to open the bathroom door. I turn the heating knob to eleven and the space is still too cold. There are two narrow single beds for some reason. Who lives in a place like this? Well, I don't. I take a peek at the map. Looks like I'm an hour's walk from anywhere. I'm hungry. I see that the Irish Emigration Museum is open and twenty-two minutes away. That will have to do.

The hotel and arena are situated in a large development in the current style – four or five storeys, black brick, autumnal-coloured steel. It could be anywhere – the US, Scandinavia, Australia. Currently it feels like a yuppie ghost town, with very few pedestrians and an indifferent wind whipping in from the west. Some St Paddy's party people reel about the blocks like little storms of gaiety, trailing silence behind them. I meet the Liffey and march along to the museum.

My greeter and ticket purveyor has been programmed to ask where I'm from. I'm welcomed as a 'Caledonian friend' and issued with a cardboard passport which I can have stamped as I weave through the exhibits. These are located in the dingy basement of the only surviving nineteenth-century warehouse hereabouts. It has been lovingly restored and barbarically repurposed. I meander through the usual video walls and interactive bollocks. I vaguely take in the ghastly statistics of the potato famine and enjoy watching a big map expand around the globe to illustrate the Irish diaspora. But much of it is the usual small-nation stuff – look how successful we've been! The Scots do it, the Welsh do it. As if we're still trying to prove to the English, we're not just peasants and cannon fodder. I told my greeter I was from Glasgow, not Scotland. Fuck nationalism, fuck patriotism. You don't get to suddenly win the world's respect because one of your country-women wrote an internationally lauded novel. You can't claim a share of an individual's achievement because you share the same nationality. What the fuck did you have to do with it?

I exit through the gift shop upstairs and take a seat under the ware-house skylights. It's a shut shopping arcade with strained pop filtering down from a tweeter somewhere in the rafters. It feels as much like Dublin as the moon. I walk into town, the throng thickening. It's not a carnival atmosphere. It's a slow, dumb drunk. In North Earl Street, a busker plays 'Whiskey in the Jar' and 'Brown Eyed Girl'. God help us all. I order a burrito in a grotty corner place with outdoor seating. The busker is competing with a bullet-headed evangelist with a headset who fortunately takes a breather as I sit down to eat. He has a banner tied to a lamppost at one end, the other end in his hand. I imagine he does this as penance. Pennants! The banner depicts diagrams illustrating the absolute certainty of getting to heaven should you follow the advertised steps. He and his colleague offer leaflets to passers-by and a surprising number accept. The tourists presumably think it's part of the festivities. The preacher pipes up again, spurting persiflage through his crappy face mic. I realise I am his only congregant. His assistant is eying me avidly. She thinks they might have hooked a sucker. I slide my eyes to the left and James Joyce's statue is squinting up into the sun. It looks like he's thinking, *Will someone shut this gobshite up?* He's an amusingly modelled figure and is striking a pose both casual and studied. The busker belts out 'Wild Mountain Thyme', the preacher squawks like a police radio and ladettes dressed as leprechauns walk by, arms linked like cancan dancers.

As I walk around, the streets fill with revellers getting into gear with their first few drinks. I swerve into the HMV store. I wonder what they sell now. Turntables and soft toys. The record players are finished in deluxe wood veneer like the radiograms our grandparents bought in the early '50s. Buy a 'vinyl' and you get a record deck for a discount. They'll be piled up in junk shops in twenty years' time. Vintage iPods will be the fashion. I take a rest on a bollard on Grattan Bridge as the tourists swarm around me. I notice the local lads have a particular hair-style – shaved at the back and sides with a moptop and a swirl of fringe. I suppose it's the *Peaky Blinders* look. They hang about McDonald's in silver tracksuits and not a stitch of emerald. The lowering sun throws long shadows across the paving. Everyone is drifting, waiting for the fun to start at the bottom of glass four. I weave through the sea of gar-ish green along the river to the east. The crowd is international and intergenerational. What exactly are they celebrating? Republicanism? Twinkle-eyed blarney? The health-giving properties of stout?

I cut through part of the big dockside development near the hotel. Signs bolted onto camera masts lay out the prohibitions: No skate-boarding, No alcohol, No food consumption. This is POPS poison – Privately Owned Public Space – with its secret rules and private policing. A group of scallywags are doing balloons of nitrous oxide. One, called Jamie, is going a bit sideways, but they're keeping an eye on him and he looks in no danger of hitting the deck. It's just that his legs have developed a mind of their own.

As I join the main drag, I'm swept into a river of the young flowing down to the 3Arena where we play tomorrow. There's an MC on tonight the kids must rate. He's BLK from Tipperary, real name Zack Walsh. I look BLK up on Wikipedia and the top hit is Blackpool Airport. Then Burgenlandkreis, a district in Saxony-Anhalt in Germany. No matter, he seems to have filled the enormodome. Maybe we should have named ourselves DLA. That's the international airport code for Douala. As I push through the crowd to the hotel, two big plainclothes cops huckle someone past, pushing his jacket over his head as if to hide his identity. Maybe it's to blind him to make escape more difficult. I walk through as if invisible. I enter the exterior glass elevator and rise like a god over the mass of people. I look down upon creation and despair of what I see.

DAY 58, Dublin, Ireland

I snap awake at 6 a.m. and squint at my blotchy pink face in the bathroom mirror as if regarding a mutilation. I watch a profoundly terrible Neil Simon comedy, *Murder by Death*, on my computer and, within ten minutes, its soporific effect takes hold. I come to at eleven. Radio 4 Extra is playing an unfunny comedy on my phone. I fumble about in the dark until I can face the glaring light of the en suite for a shave. Gavin is not helpful when shaving. One has to rush each scrape to counter any lateral deviations. One serious sideways wobble and you're slit like an avocado. But the first pill has taken hold and all is reasonably steady. I imagine having a carer shave me and wish to be dead before such a thing is necessary. When we came down from the high dais in Manchester, we passed two local crew guys with enormous beards standing side by side. For some preposterous reason, I motioned with my hand as if cupping my own invisible beard, as if two big-bearded guys were an extraordinarily rare sight. One grinned and the other frowned. I mean, you wouldn't do the same with breasts, would you? I'm not embarrassed. I'm happy to understand that this makes me an old fool.

I pull my wheeled luggage the fifty yards from hotel to arena. I walk around the wide circle made by the back of the bleachers and find a lift to our dressing area. We have four rooms with frosted-glass windows running along the wall at head height, so you have a vague sense of an outside world.

Today I am to be interviewed by old journalist acquaintance Craig McLean for the third and final bit of media we decided I'd do around my public outing as a Parkinson's person. As with the radio show and Laura Kuenssberg chat, I'm nervous about doing it. Talking about music is easy. Talking about life is hard. It does not come naturally when you've spent your life scrupulously avoiding discussing your personal life in public. I sort of sleepwalked into coming out in the media about the Ghastly Affliction. After hiding it for so long while my mother was alive, her typically elegant and polite death left me in limbo. I was free to be open, but uncertain about stepping out of the anonymity of keeping my diagnosis within a tight circle of friends and family. I knew it had to be done, but did not consider what impact, if any, disclosure would have.

I was caught off guard when a Canadian news agency published as a 'story' the advance programme details from the BBC Radio 4 documentary I'd taken part in on the subject. It never occurred to me it would be in any way 'news'. Suddenly, I was inundated with messages. As the radio show had yet to be broadcast, I just took cover, removed myself from social media and haven't been back since. That sabbatical has been a great relief. I wanted to let the interviews speak for themselves. Our manager, Andy P (an experienced press agent), had eased me so gently into the whole process that I was hardly aware of anything particularly noteworthy happening. There were a few approaches from Scottish newspapers, which I politely declined. I didn't wish such a minor matter to be overstated. As a story, it mattered only to a small group of people.

Craig and I hug hello. He's been interviewing us since his first forays into music journalism, starting out writing for Scottish free sheets and going on to become deputy editor of the *Face* and contributing regularly to major publications. Today, he's talking to me for *The Times*. I've always liked Craig and we reminisce for a few minutes about various drunken evenings before eliding seamlessly into the interview. I tell him that his piece about Beck for the *Face* in the mid-'90s was my favourite bit of music writing of the era. He makes talking about the Ghastly Affliction easy. He tells me his father was a P person too, so he knows what to ask about and, gratifyingly, knows how real it is, despite appearances. I do a photo shoot with local snapper Johnny Savage who doesn't fuck about and takes some lovely frames outside at the end of the session. Seeing any photo of me not looking stricken is a tonic for my soul. Thanks, Johnny.

I'm late taking pill two, but feel fine and decide not to take a third until after our show. The arena bellows and resounds with an absurd din during the soundcheck. These places all sound like you're playing at the bottom of a mine shaft on the far side of a canyon. They're brutal acoustic environments. They're the aural equivalent of hanging an art exhibition on a cliff face that is only accessible by helicopter. You peer out of your moving window to dimly discern a picture. You think it's Whistler's *Arrangement in Grey and Black No. 1*, but you can't be 100 per cent certain. It might be a seagull nest.

In catering, I sit and chat with Gordon Goudie, the Minds' second guitarist of the last seven or so years. Gordon has played with Echo & the Bunnymen and we sing the praises of *Ocean Rain*, their fourth album masterpiece. He tells me a few tales. I know Ian McCulloch can be a handful, but I adore him, and Mac and Gordon obviously have a great relationship. He's one of the great post-'70s English male rock singers, along with Richard Ashcroft and Liam Gallagher. And, like Edwyn Collins, he's never been afraid to slag off other acts he regards as inferior. I love that – it's so anti-showbiz. And it's brave. You never know when you might bump into artists you've denigrated. And they may have security.

Iain and I watch the Minds' big intro from stage right. They start with the awesome, enormous 'Waterfront'. The bass swings – dum-de-dum-de-dum – and you wait for that massive pair of chord stabs. When they come in, Iain and I turn to one another and burst out laughing. It's so ridiculous, so enthralling. It's why rock music can be such amazing fun. Back in 1989, when we scaled up from clubs to the Pavilion Theatre in Glasgow, we thought it deserved marking with a statement, so we performed a medley of Scottish pop – Orange Juice's 'Blue Boy' and Simple Minds' 'Waterfront', topped off with 'Shang-A-Lang' by the Bay City Rollers. I remember my mother, up in a box an arm's length from stage right, looking thrilled and relieved we'd pulled off a sold-out theatre show. We booked wedding car limos to take us to the after-show party. Everything was a fucking hoot.

DAY 59, Belfast, UK

Another day, another dockside development. Ten storeys of balconied apartments stand where shipyards used to churn out tonnage. Yes, there is black brick; yes, the balcony balustrades are chrome and glass.

I'm walking to the Titanic museum in the sharp sunlight and bitter air. I pay my £24.95 at ticket booth one. The price is not a good start. The building, on the approach, is completely hideous, like an abstracted hedgehog. When a building resembles anything other than a building, it's a failure. Architecture is the art of engineering, not the engineering of art. I start at the Galley café with a decent coffee and a Chelsea bun that tastes like it's been sweating in its polythene packaging since the *Titanic* launched. I look through a wall of glass onto a construction site where a concrete mixer turns surprisingly rapidly and an enormous corkscrew is pulled out of the ground. They're still making shit, you have to admit. It's probably going to be a museum dedicated to the building of this museum.

For those who will never visit the Titanic museum, here's the gist: they built a big boat in Belfast, it hit a berg and went down. You already know all the maiden-voyage-unsinkable-opulent-hubris stuff. It's not a complicated story with complicated meanings. It nicely foreshadows the Great War, and it speaks to both the survival advantages conferred by wealth and status and their futility. That's why Bob Dylan invokes the *Titanic* at least twice, why so many films have been made, why Beryl Bainbridge wrote *Every Man for Himself*. You just don't need a fucking museum. The whole exhibition functions like a ghost train. You're pumped up to the top of the ride to spiral back down to earth through eerie imagery accompanied by spooky music. There's a large video wall display listing the names of all the lost and all the saved, which has a smidgeon of poetry about it. But apart from the symbolism of nature trumping human ingenuity, the sinking of the *Titanic* is insignificant compared to the cataclysmic waste of human life everywhere else in the twentieth century. But I get it – the moonless night, the millpond, the rich in first class and the poor in steerage, the band playing on, the porthole lights slipping under – the story is seamed with pristine narrative imagery like a fairy tale manufactured in a steel furnace.

I walk around the old dry docks, past the giant yellow goalposts of Harland & Wolff's Samson and Goliath cranes, to a pedestrian bridge over the Lagan. I'm reminded of Cleveland – all this heavy maritime industry so near town. I stop at a big tourist information map. Someone has seen the good sense to adorn a photograph of Queen Victoria with a pair of bushy eyebrows and a moustache, finished off with a cock and balls poking at her right cheek. As always, she looks unamused. In fact, she looks furious.

In town on the far side of the river, I rifle through the three tiny floors of Young Savage Vintage – the usual ugly leathers, synthetic knitwear and faded T-shirts you find the world over. The books on the top floor are better curated, but I feel no urge. I have lunch in the courtyard of a boutique hotel called Bullitt. The weather is on the cusp between mild spring and the last icy licks of winter. I meander into the same square I sat in two years ago. I check my blog from 2022. Back then, there was Jelvis the Pelvis plying his trade. Today, a young busker plays pop hits until he is drowned out by a deafening Christian with a much louder speaker. The busker gamely fights back. It's open war. The god botherer is from the Church of Jesus Christ, whom I can only assume are cunts if this guy is anything to go by. He's intoning at the top of his lungs outside a shop called White Stuff. His spiel is hectoring and enervating. Busker boy hits back with 'Wonderwall'. I drop him a note in his guitar case to show some secular solidarity. He says I'm much too kind and I give him a wink. We must stand firm against the tyranny of the righteous.

I find a single copy of Del Amitri's *Fatal Mistakes* for £6.99 in the HMV CD racks. So, we still have a stake in the culture. Just. I'm now desperately trying to kill time before returning to the dim environment of the arena. I walk through an upmarket arcade of the new type – an open-ended 'street' with an airport-type roof, café seating down the middle. I have a coffee-chain beverage under an awning and watch the people amble by. You would never know there was an unacknowledged civil war raging here thirty years ago. A man called Gary crosses the street to shake my hand. He's incredibly kind and gracious. I'm a stranger here. I'm a lucky man.

The venue is pretty horrible. Used for ice hockey in winter, it's a vast black fridge. Our dressing room is a big cold locker room and smells strongly of Deep Heat. No wonder hockey players get so wound up – their working environment is vile. It sounds like shit. I hide on the bus between soundcheck and our 7.15 showtime. The ice under the venue floor makes your feet cold. You cannot relax if you have cold feet.

I forget to take my third pill and it preys on my mind during the show. I feel my right hand stiffening as the 3 p.m. dose wears off. I have to readjust my plectrum a few times, my grip relaxing instead of my wrist. Of course, I suspect this is purely psychological rather than pharmacological. But popping the third dose gives my confidence a boost. I take to the bus straight after, listening to music in the back lounge and scarfing chocolate. Long drive to London tonight and a 3 a.m. ferry crossing. We move by night, we circus creatures, and we come quietly at dawn.

DAY 60, London, UK

I shove up the concertina blinds on the bus staircase to see the scrag end of the Lake District floating by. I sit on the top step for a gaze when the second driver appears for the day shift. He's clutching an armful of sugar and caffeine products. I estimate we're six hours from our hotel.

I dive back into my bunk, swapping the slumber-inducing drone of Eric Hobsbawm's *The Age of Revolution* for the bracing, manic exhortations of Bob Dylan's *Saved*. I ease into my morning routine. *Guardian* Quick Crossword, *New York Times* Wordle, Mini Crossword, Connections and finally Spelling Bee, which takes the rest of the day to complete. I flop out of my slot around half-eleven, regarding the fields of England swimming in mist. It doesn't look like today will ever get started. The sky is so low you can feel it in your hair. We're east of Liverpool, north of Crewe, sailing slowly south, all colour wrung out of the world. I debate whether to put on my shoes. I feel I need a bus kilt – something casual and cool to lounge around in. I go downstairs for a coffee. Jim and Andy are swapping rock tales with Simon the driver. We pull in for a toilet stop, three identically liveried Phoenix buses parked in a row. Convoy!

We draw into London after four, the two thickets of skyline silhouetted in a silty light with an armada of battleship clouds serried out to the channel. We're on the North Circular, as ugly an approach to a capital city as you'll find anywhere in the world. The Shard, the Walkie-Talkie and the Cheese Grater lean around in a style-less sulk, while off to the east, the more monumental edifices at Canary Wharf stand straight and blank-faced like a wall of riot police. Mr Fudge informs us that our rooms have been upgraded. We schlep along a corridor to a separate tower where I take a private elevator to find my lavishly appointed suite surrounded on three sides by men in hard hats. Their heads are at roughly knee height, and they seem keen to ignore me, beetling about on their platforms suspended fifty feet above the tarmac. The outside of our tower is still being clad it would appear. I open my heavy balcony door to say hello to one of the builders, but he scurries away. We're in the Intercontinental, which is attached to the O2, or as I know it, the Millennium Dome, one of the big infrastructure projects closely associated with the Blair administration. It's a temple to New Labour – flashy, privately owned, repurposed and shop-soiled, like Tony himself.

The whole venue complex sits secured behind a blue mesh fence and I have to do a bit of a detour to get to the river path that runs around the rim of the Greenwich Peninsula. The river here has a faint scent of the sea and laps at the sandy banks like an ocean meeting a beach. I look to the Isle of Dogs on the opposite bank, the office lights in the towers starting to glow as the sun sets behind. Gulls squeal and laugh beneath a line of landing jets. Four fat geese flap past with a muted honk. I walk on, the river widening, a high three-quarter moon bald as an eye above. I come to Antony Gormley's *Quantum Cloud*, inelegantly plonked on its four-legged platform like an exploding Easter egg. The river smells of shit. I walk by the giant towers of the IFS Cloud Cable Car. This is all new to me, a different London.

I come to a junction that affords me access to the Dome area and find a noodle chain place to park myself and refuel. There's a wait in spite of the many free tables and I figure they're short staffed. I'm led to a stool at a counter facing a window and reckon getting fed might take a while. The room is filled with the confident noise Londoners make when they're out and loud. Darkness falls beyond the glass and the reflection of the diners behind me floats in the same plane as the passers by outside. Even in a mid-price joint like this, the wealth is conspicuous. Compared to Glasgow or any backwater – Middlesbrough, Stoke, Swansea – the clothes, the bags, the hair and cologne... It's all just a bit more expensive. You can smell the money. It whispers like a taunt.

I complete the full circuit around the Dome, angling across the concourse as graceful kids reel around on roller skates like slender giants.

DAY 61, London, UK

I pick up where I left off last night and walk down the eastern side of the peninsula until the Thames Barrier comes into view. It's as if somebody has dismantled Sydney Opera House and strung it across the river. The waterside infrastructure down here is all dilapidated piers and hulks of filthy barges anchored on rusty chains. The planes whine under the roof of low cloud, the sun suddenly warm on my back in random patches.

I come upon two Scottish women emerging from an ecology park looking for a café. I wander in along wooden walkways and sit in the bird hide under a canopy of cobwebs. There's a blackboard on the wall where spotters have chalked up their sightings. I'm tempted to write 'fat bird', but remind myself this is not funny. Big bird. That's funny. On the way out, I fondle some pussy willow, its furred flesh exquisite to the touch. Phwoar. In the gatehouse, I make a donation. I'm all heart, me. The woolly man who thanks me looks so like one's idea of an ecologist he might have been knitted for a gift shop. Back on the Thames Path, I come across a lost moorhen darting about in a panic, separated from the wetland by a yacht club. I look down on a dun-coloured beach, the waves leaving deposits of inky soot upon it like lines of text.

The path leads through the Tarmac Aggregates plant. Metal track-ways fly overhead, conveying product to river transportation. There's a giant pyramid of sand and just beyond that the Anchor & Hope, a quaint pub with a beer garden facing the water. I take my place at a picnic table, a lone sobrietist amongst a gaggle of boozers, all nattering in those big, wide London vowels. It's lovely. I look back at the city, its flurry of towers, pecked and picked at by a flock of cranes.

Past the barrier, I stop at a bench opposite the huge Tate & Lyle sugar factory, which is noisily venting a plume of white steam. The river here looks deeper, the surface marbled with channels and eddies. There's a man with an easel on the path. I wonder if I'm sullying his composition. He's doing that thing of holding his brush between his eye and the horizon. Maybe he's trying to block me out. As I walk by him, I discover I'm at the end of the trail, so have to about-face and pass him again. He's made a few charcoal marks; not bad, not bad, I think. On the two-mile walk back, I see Damien Hirst's *The Mermaid*, some sort of irony-heavy parody of shopping mall art which I do not understand. I've seen the shark with the pretentious title and thought it very impressive, evocative of some terrible loneliness. This statue is a turd in a raincoat.

After a remarkably pain-free show, our dressing room is suddenly flooded with guests as we're still changing out of our stage clobber. I fix a couple of drinks for people and slide out. I cannot hack the bon-homie, the fraternising, the shooting of the breeze. It sends me into a strange mixture of panic and torpor. I hide on the bus in the upstairs back lounge and read some *Private Eye* and *Viz* to calm down. I very much want to go to bed, but there's a guest, Trisha Reid, I'd like to catch up with after the Minds. Trisha was in a Glasgow band called Sophisticated Boom Boom (later His Latest Flame) who were the only all-female group of the early '80s in Scotland that mattered, along with the duo Strawberry Switchblade. Del Amitri became friendly with them around 1986–87, Iain going out with Trisha and I with drummer Jacquie. It was incredibly enlightening hearing how these women got through the same shitty support tours and record company hassles we'd endured. In some ways, everything was differ-ent for the girls, but in most ways, everything was the same. The two bands lifted each other's morale, sharing rehearsal space and forming a party band that morphed into a country outfit called Sadie Bagwash & Cowpoke. The women in His Latest Flame helped us, advised us and made us feel like we weren't going mad. They were our sisters. Trisha, especially, along with her brother Ian, taught us a lot about Hank Williams and the dark side of the Celtic soul. There's a strain of Irish lyricism that gets curdled like gassed milk in Glasgow Catholic culture. Without it, we'd be nothing.

We leave London at 1 a.m., red lights on the cranes, a high moon, the river shining and serpentine. It's all so amazing while they're still building it. It'll be a disaster when they finish.

DAY 62, Birmingham, UK

Our credit card-style hotel keys are in our hands at 10 a.m., so off the bus we go and up we all scoot in the lift with our wheeled trunks. I head straight out for breakfast, finding Iain in a local caff and joining him at a tight little table by the door. Two forty-something men come in as we're finishing our meals and request a photo. They're very charming, so I forgive the interruption of our repast. For some godforsaken reason, they're going to watch Arbroath vs Partick Thistle tomorrow (because they liked the look of the ground they say). They're both very likeable, open people and I imagine they're going to have a great time. I weave uphill to Birmingham Museum & Art Gallery, coming across another Antony Gormley – *Iron:Man*, a rusted four-metre-high figure bound by a cross of steel. He looks like a burial at sea bobbing up through the concrete. It's my third Gormley of the tour. That tells you more about how successful he is at winning commissions than the quality of his work, most of which revolves around representations of himself as some sort of post-industrial superhero. I bump into Andy who is also stuck for something to do. It's cold, there's nowt on at the flicks and half the public museum is shut for renovation.

A tall young man approaches, commenting on my hair, offering me a free haircut. He hands me a card. If I present it at Shepherds on New Street, I get a 'complimentary service'. Do I look unkempt? Last time I checked, I thought I was reasonably kempt. His boss must have booted him into the street this morning: *Go get me some old guys with long hair.* I pay £11 to see 'Victorian Radicals', a motley collection of Pre-Raphaelite and Arts and Crafts stuff, mainly paintings of languid girls with lustrous curls and lantern jaws. The gallery is teeming with retired fuckers, milling about stupidly and butting in front of your view. I'm like them. We're brain-dead cunts. We've sucked the light out of the world and we're fucking off into hell with it and you're not getting it back. Broom! Broom! We're all just killing time before the real killing begins. In my case, it has already started. I hate what I'm becoming. I leave the exhibition and notice its venue – Gas Hall. Gas us all. Gas us all to hell.

I drift into a shopping mall, the chill in the air a bit too sharp for relaxation. I take coffee and a big biscuit from a young, reticent barista working within an island on the concourse. He's gorgeous but I don't think he likes to be thought of that way. His geeky friend drops by, calls him Bro' and tries to get a conversation going about a video game. But the barista has customers to take care of, the females of whom are seriously giving him the eye. He flirts back unthreateningly, hating himself. I'm losing the will to go on wandering. I decide to take the afternoon off. Up in my seventh-floor box, I float on my luxury mattress to Alice Coltrane's lofty harp at Carnegie Hall. From my bed, I can see the British School and the back of Singers Hill Synagogue, the loveliest collection of syllables I've seen all day.

Sleep washes over me, the delicious sloth of a stolen afternoon. Iain messages to say he has blagged tickets for The Smile. We meet at eight, along with Gavin (the man, not the trembling hand) and walk down the hill to the venue. We know we've played here but can't remember when. We try the balcony, order enormous two-pint beers (mine, sadly, sans alcohol) and attempt to find a decent viewing pitch, standing behind blokes who are standing behind the seats. Thom Yorke is completely invisible, as is the reed player, so we content ourselves with watching Jonny Greenwood and the drummer, Tom Skinner. Iain makes it to the opposite side where he can see the other half of the stage. Me and Gav navigate the tricky route along the narrow gangway at the back of the balcony, apologising to everyone we squeeze past in turn. I manage to catch a few glimpses of Yorke between two heads. He has a pleasing intensity. I half-dance to a couple of odd-time grooves. It's exactly what I expected. It reminds me a little of the magnificent BEAK>, also a supergroup of sorts. I last less than an hour before I make my excuses. I need food. I have a thali in a nearby modern curry house. The waitress is savagely good at her job and the food is fucking delicious. All in all, it's been a brilliant day off. I feel lucky as fuck.

DAY 63, Birmingham, UK

Ablutions. Some stretches, a shave and the White Album. This is the record where Paul does pastiche and Lennon does super weird. 'Bungalow Bill' is the best anti-war song I know. The opening lyrics of 'Happiness is a Warm Gun' are deranged. The album is peak-Lennon – twisted, angry, disgusted and sarcastic. Macca seems cornered, running for the safety of parody, tweeness and triteness, until 'Helter Skelter' when he has a magnificent nervous breakdown. It's the first time I've listened to it sober for a few years. It still frightens me.

It's a short ride on the bus from hotel to venue. I munch some healthy grub in catering and attempt a walk. Five minutes in and I'm hit by a hailstorm. Everything is suddenly unpleasant. I have a feel-ing the sun will be out in an hour, so I take shelter back at the gig in another sports changing area dressing room, all hose-down blue Formica and grey tiles. At least there's heating. Jim Kerr has warned us that Nottingham, like the Belfast venue, does ice hockey, so it'll be another giant freezer. That's the thing you always forget about the British spring – there are many false dawns. You have a warm clement day and you think you've made it when winter comes howling back the following morning.

I'm proved right. I peek out of the fire doors around 1 p.m. and it's sunny. I stroll out aimlessly, bumping into Andrew, an Oxford friend of Iain's, who shot some lovely photos of the band at Barrowland in 2018. We have a chat on Broad Street in the piercing light and wind. I sense Andrew might be appalled at the ravages the six years have wrought. 2018 is a different world: pre-Covid, pre-diagnosis, pre-stroke. I glanced in the toilet mirror today and the wreck staring back was both frightened and frightening. Frightful, in fucking fact. After fifty-five, it's good light or goodnight. I push my frame into a coffee shop to rest my feet. The long walk in Greenwich has wearied me. I can't get into rhythm, I'm yet to hit my stride. Gavin shakes his little reminder at my side, my loving, faithful com-panion. Iain comes into the café and doesn't see me. I wave in a wide, desperate arc 'til he spots me. We sit in companionable silence, pot-tering at our devices.

Back at the arena, I enter via the front door, getting caught up in the VIP queue for the Minds' soundcheck party. A few folk grab me for photos, for which I pose awkwardly, feeling a bit trapped. I take a seat towards the back of the enormous space as the punters file in below me. I talk to a staff member who is checking all the rows for obstructions and trip hazards. She says it takes three hours.

I can't figure out how they've managed to fit this huge barn in the middle of Birmingham. The Minds enter to the effusive cheers of the four hundred gold ticket holders. Jim does his usual spiel, peppered with off-the-cuff stuff. Again, he's so relaxed, the epitome of a man comfortable in his own skin. 'I Travel' gets them on their feet. Jim does a comedy spoken-word bit in the middle referencing a Celtic player on loan at West Bromwich Albion, a local club. It's all perfectly pitched between shtick and sentiment. I can't help but be charmed by them.

Ours is the best show so far, according to the band. I try not to kill the vibe, but feel it incumbent on me not to lie. I can't fake the glee. I spent the whole set at war with the Ghastly Affliction. I couldn't get my plectrum in a proper grip, and I felt like my arm was seizing up. I struggled with my singing, which felt strange in my throat, like I was driving a car wearing flippers and boxing gloves. At times like these, a voice in my head keeps hissing: *you've got to stop, you've got to stop.* That's not fun to contend with in front of six thousand people. I'm just glad to get out alive.

A friend from Glasgow sends a picture of me that his mate took in Birmingham. I look like a rock god. I look like a scarecrow.

DAY 64, Nottingham, UK

I'm awake in my bunk at dawn, but work hard on getting back under. Next stop midday. A good long rest. Will that keep the extreme shakes at bay? The sun is spilling around the grim loading area. I make for Rough Trade and browse the music biography table, eschewing a Prince tome for a Simple Minds book called *Themes for Great Cities*. A fiver! Outside, there's a queue of moderately gothy-looking youth forming for an instore signing. I have a veggie breakfast in a corner café next door. The staff are all about seventeen, the customers young college students. I am pleasingly invisible. I can study them without anyone catching my gaze, so involved are they in their discourse. It's deeply relaxing to be so unseen. My life is a film without principal characters, only background noise and room tone for a soundtrack.

Nottingham is an attractive little city, less damaged by the Luftwaffe than Birmingham. It has all you'd want from a city in miniature. A bit of urban decay, a bit of gentrification, a bit of grime and a bit of glitz, and enough historical fabric intact to be quaint. I traipse about sluggishly trying to mop up the occasional shaft of sunlight slanting through a back lane. I find myself in a Waterstones. I've not been reading recently – no focus, no concentration. My mother was book-mad and I miss her recommendations. I look at ten things that don't grab me until I open a Jim Thompson book called *Pop. 1280*. Psycho sheriff, unreliable narrator. That looks right for my current mood.

I have a decent show, less tortured than last night by the nagging voices of doom. Besides, it's a decent-sounding room for an arena. We scarper for the tour bus at 9.15, Jim and I only catching half an hour of the Minds' set. We're disappointed about having to leave – they're sounding good in this smaller space. We get into our Bournemouth hotel at two in the morning and are quickly issued with keys by a couple of friendly night porters, the elder of whom kindly helps me with the lift. My room is mad, a big elliptical sweep of floor-to-ceiling windows, a lounge, double bedroom and two bathrooms. There's room for two armchairs, a ten-seater sofa, a dining table with four chairs and two enormous televisions. In the morning, I find a wind-blasted balcony running round the whole suite. I feel like I'm in an apartment in the Watergate building. I make a coffee and luxuriate. One of the joys of touring is the unexpected treats like this. I don't want to leave. What joys could Bournemouth possibly have in store to compete with this?

DAY 65, day off, Bournemouth, UK

I lounge in my enormous suite, peering at the map for inspiration. A search for 'art gallery' yields a bunch of shitty shops selling tat. 'Attractions' pulls up a pier, an oceanarium and an upside-down house. I think it will have to be beach and lunch.

I'm at the seafront in minutes and buy a ticket for a big wheel. I'm the only customer. My gondola arcs upwards to the apex and I look down on six labourers in orange hi-vis suits swabbing the concourse with stiff brushes and a high-pressure hose. There's a sign above the bench seat with the usual proscriptions – No Drinking, No Smoking, but also No Punching Windows. And No Kicking Windows. Gosh, I wish someone had told me years ago – I wouldn't have all these scars. The wheel does three or four turns. It's not much of a view, beach stretching in both directions, a jumble of town facing a blank sea. People are milling about looking vaguely at leisure. The white sunlight is splashing about under a thin quilt.

I make for the aquarium, buying a ticket from an encouragingly happy girl at the counter. I take a spiral staircase up to the exhibits, past a staff member sweeping sand into little piles at the side of each step. At the top, I'm greeted by a green iguana, who's very pretty with his gold sequinned arms and all-body Mohican, but could easily be a plastic toy for all he's performing. I think he's looking at me, but could be looking beyond me, imagining better places, better times. He's on a shelf in a greenhouse that's made up like some tropical beach hut. It's all redolent of an '80s nightclub in Carlisle. In a darkened corridor, I'm confronted by a column of piranha, loitering disinterestedly like little bruisers waiting for a ruck. They're a brick of muscle with thuggish lips and vacant eyes. Opposite this tank of cunts are some huge red pacu who've evolved human-like teeth to crush nuts and seeds. There is a smattering of catfish among them and a big ray whose polka-dot back would make a fine pattern for a cravat. These are all Amazon dwellers. The idea of wading in a muddy river with such bulky creatures gives me the fear. Looking at fish reputedly lowers one's heart rate and I feel curiously somnambulant gazing into these graceful animals' secret world.

Just beyond is a pretty, petite turtle I admire until suddenly cornered by buggies and kids. I'm in another pram jam, cornered like a rat. I have to 'excuse me' my way out, the rudest phrase in the language. There's no action in the otter pen. They have a pool and a playground full of green, blue and pink balls, but nothing's doing. I finally locate two curled up cutely together in a corner like ying and yang. There's more activity among the zebra cichlids and featherfin catfish, who are all darting about like fireworks. I am trapped in the snarl of pushchairs again and try to wait for them to pass through, but they linger and block all movement along the passageways.

I spot a door marked Bay View Terrace Café and slip onto a little indoor deck with tables and chairs and a wall of glass looking out to sea. I am in a human display case. No one has come to see us today. A young couple at a nearby table are listening to a voicemail on speakerphone. It's so long that the girl says 'it's like listening to a podcast'. Some sizeable waves are breaking with a crump, the contrast between the mustard sand and pale green water pleasing to the eye. A few hardy sorts are braving the wind, their toddlers mucking about with bucket and spade and waddling into the surf. A video display on the pier advertises Badness, a Madness tribute band who are playing Fathers' Day weekend. The odd thing about the south coast is that the closer you get to France, the more resolutely English everything gets – flags of St George everywhere, fish and chips, floral gardens, beer gardens, garden gnomes. Like they're all giving Europe the vicky – morris dancing and scoffing roast beef and warm bitter.

I rejoin the route, looking down into a large pool of circling sharks and a massive turtle the size of a car. A keeper feeds the creature Chinese lettuce with a grabber stick, but when she introduces seafood, the other little fish come speeding in to steal the bounty. The keeper gives the turtle's back a scrape and it moons off lugubriously. It's an awesome beast. Putting her in a tank the size of a squash court is like putting a horse in a matchbox; it makes no sense. I check with the keeper and I'm right about the turtle's sex and omnivorousness. She eats mainly fish, I'm told. In another room, a small lone penguin swoops about like an underwater comet behind a big glass screen. He swims like he's flying and looks disturbed by the limits of his world. There's a creepy section called the Abyss featuring critters from the deep, with very low light and glass domes you stick your head up into to see crabs spidering about inches from your nose. Ominous music plays. It's very trippy and it makes Gavin tremble. Beyond is the unfortunately named spotted scat, bunked up with an elusive electric eel. I spot a comical grey fish with a cartoon nose, but fail to find his details. He looks like a Dickens lawyer running late for a case.

I march back uphill to the penthouse bar in the hotel to catch Marco Rossi, Jim's old bandmate from the Kevin McDermott Orchestra, visiting from Weymouth. Marco is a guitar god, one of Greenock's most legendary musical sons. He's the musician's musician to many – modest, sublimely skilful and as happy to play in a pub doing obscure NRBQ covers as perform in arenas as a session player. We chat about the Left Banke and another Greenock maestro, George Miller of the Kaisers, the note- and stitch-perfect '60s beat combo I blagged to play at Iain's wedding. It's still one of the best gigs I've seen.

I sip some double-zero Italian lager with them both until hunger starts to distract. Back down on the esplanade, I take tea in a Harry Ramsden's, the bogus-authentic chip shop chain. The waiter is a comedy-camp 1970s sitcom character with tartan specs, male pattern baldness and a diseased right eye. He keeps the old ladies entertained, but when he starts throwing chairs around while resetting tables, I want to throttle him. I look out through the fake stained-glass windows on my fake art deco chair on a fake parquet floor. The sea is still green, the sand a warm beige. 'Ticket to Ride' comes spilling from lo-fi ceiling speakers. Perhaps the corporate music supply cunts consider it a seaside selection because it contains the word 'ride'. I can see the Isle of Wight. I'm full of carbs and coffee. I'm a touring bloke, beached in Bournemouth.

Marco had told us there's a bit of a county lines problem here and, after a brisk sojourn along the front, I wind up the hill into town to encounter a far more edgy locale than the promenade. A guy tries to accost me with a sob story about being in the army and quickly gets shirty when I don't stop to listen to him. A young woman advises me to say 'Ola!' next time – 'then they think you don't understand them'. It all starts kicking off in a Tesco round the corner. The duty manager and a young security guard are trying to get a nutcase to leave with, it has to be said, very careful physical contact. The guy stands protesting on the threshold and, as I approach, he ejects a shaft of saliva forcing me into a surprisingly agile sidestep. I, pointlessly, ask the security guy if he's going to be alright. What the fuck am I going to do? Sing a song? Retirees, Brexiteers and hard drugs – what a weird town.

DAY 66, Bournemouth, UK

Farewell Watergate suites. The venue is next door to the hotel, but we get on the bus anyway. I'm last off and can't find an in, so give up and go walking in sporadic pinpricks of rain. I ascend some steep steps, finding nothing but a car park at their summit. I peruse a tourist map on a large piece of signage. Not a clue. I meander down again through a wooded churchyard, popping into the church itself for about thirty seconds of profound serenity, in the side, out the front. How do churches do this, the instant hush, the sharp shutting-out of the corporeal world? It's the neatest trick in religion's box.

I spot a breakfast blackboard outside a tapas place and am seated by a very smiley woman whose husband is sweating and sighing behind the hot lamps. My toast comes on a weird little dish designed for corn on the cob, so I have to hold the slices in the flat palm of my left hand and spread the butter with my right. This is a military operation for me. That's the disease – the slow death of dexterity. The food cheers me. I've been in a foul mood. Iain messaged me last night to let me know our long-ailing friend Jaine Henderson is being 'made comfortable' in hospital. I've just been reading about Jaine in the Simple Minds book I bought in Nottingham.

Jaine and her brother David were involved at an early stage with the group, operating their lighting and sound desks respectively. David was our go-to soundman for many years. They're tall, gentle, incredibly stylish people who, along with their mother Mary, have been fixtures on the Glasgow gig scene for as long as I can remember. Iain and I had visited Jaine in hospital shortly before we started the tour and, coincidentally, Andy had turned up at the same time. It was a lovely afternoon. I spent five months visiting My Love in the same hospital in 2023. I never want to go there again. I think of Jaine and just hope she's not in pain. We are now on tenterhooks. I watch the couple running the tapas bar and think of friends Matty and Claire who run a similar-sized operation in Glasgow, up at dawn six days a week, slinging panini and homemade soup at a queue of office grafters. I admire hard work, but these days I'm hard pushed to remember what it's like. I work less than a two-hour day. Everything is winding down. Everything must go.

It's still spitting outside so I get coffee in Blend, one of those metro-sexual anti-Starbucks coffee houses where everyone is tapping at a laptop and wearing clothes bought from the same online store as that wanker who owns Facebook. I slump into a low chair as overdesigned as it is uncomfortable. The other customers are pretending they're working from home, but I suspect they're cruising chat forums under assumed identities after getting ChatGPT 4 to fill out their recent job applications. The music sounds like Morrissey moaning from the bottom of a well. Shazam tells me it's Khruangbin & Leon Bridges, a record I thought I knew. It's so hard to get new memories to stick. Life used to supply a torrent of events that were quickly imprinted onto the chip. Now it's a wilderness of nothing, punctuated by rare flashes of something random. Why does one particular memory, of all the other possible memories, get saved? If I don't write it down by next week, it won't exist.

The café is located in the old art deco *Evening Echo* newspaper building, a high-ceilinged space that once must have hummed with activity, mechanical and human. Now it's chill-out tunes and the soft shuffle of fingers scraping at track pads. I leave to look for a quiet place to make a phone call and find myself in another church, this time Catholic; the same hush, the same sepulchral air. For reasons someone has to explain to me, all the statues have been completely covered by purple drapes as if suddenly considered obscene. It must be 'hide your saints' day.

My friend Geoff picks me up around 3.30 and we go to chi-chi Sandbanks, taking a pot of tea in a Rick Stein gaff. Someone goes by in a blacked-out Bentley. How vulgar, I think. It's nice to get out beyond the circus encampment for an hour. There's an open fire and we swap stories about our parents dying and our illnesses, the usual things people of our age talk about. Right now, I cannot see a future for me and I panic every time I contemplate it. Idle thoughts of suicide passed through my mind on stage. The thought of achieving death is the last comfort, the one state of being that can stop all this rubbish. Not being. It's a fantasy that keeps me from true despair.

DAY 67, Cardiff, UK

I pill up at midday and get some lunch in catering. On venturing forth, I find myself re-treading the same steps as 2021. It's inevitable. Unless you plot a specific route to a specific destination, you are condemned to repeat ad infinitum. The arcades, the high street, the castle. The same indoor market with the same shit record shop and shit mod shirt shop. In the pedestrianised centre, I pass some Christians warbling about love or some such, one propped up on a life-size cross. They're fighting with the Wurlitzer organ from a nearby carousel.

It's windy and a bit damp. I'm waiting for ex-Dels guitarist Dave Cummings to arrive from London. Dave is the eldest of five brothers, sons of Irish parents from Crawley. On joining the group in 1989, Dave took on a big brother/scout leader role. He'd cajole us into playing parlour games, going out to baseball matches, comedy shows, building bonfires on the beach. So many of our happiest memories of that era are a consequence of some plan Dave had instigated. When he hung out with his mates in Madness before we'd met, they nicknamed him Mad Dog because he was always so sensible and grown up about how to have fun. He was missed when he retired in 1996, off to start a family and a career in screenwriting. I think his fantastic playing on *Twisted* is a perfect legacy.

I meet Dave around four in Corner Coffee on the high street with his friend Abi, an actor/producer from Paisley whose parents were from Wales. Dave tells me she had a cardiac arrest a while back.

Later in the dressing room, Abi says she had a torn aorta (I think) and was bedridden for months. She lives with the knowledge that this could reoccur at any moment. Before the show, Andy told me that his ex-girlfriend just lost her daughter to a heart attack four days ago. Death is everywhere. The young, the old – none of us are safe, all in peril.

The bus pulls us north through the rain. I have 'Fall in Love With Me' by Iggy Pop on the stereo. The mint-green LED light strips in the ceiling make the back lounge feel like a little nightclub. I'm high above the road in a box of colour and noise, a moving point of hope in all the blackness.

DAY 68, day off, Glasgow, UK

We're in the truck park alongside the Hydro, the hometown arena we headlined in 2014. I'm up at half-eleven, last off the bus. I expect most are at the funeral of rehearsal complex owner Steve Cheyne. I taxi the short trip home and spend an hour catching up with Luke, My Love's lovely son who's been kindly housesitting again and doing cat maintenance. He's been dealing with all the serious shit while I've been gone and I'm humbled with gratitude. I get on my bike and am in the nursing home at two.

The staff are transferring My Love to bed. She has a lot of issues with pain and often asks to be put into her bed in the afternoons. It always feels more normal to talk to her when she is in her wheelchair, on the same level, face to face, cheek to cheek. We can dovetail like two drivers facing opposite directions, window to window, side by side. In bed, it's more of a medical situation. The second thing she says is 'I've got to get out of here'. My heart turns to liquid and drains from my chest. As the staff get her into the hoist, I sit in the empty lounge, normally abuzz with carers and residents, TV blaring, tea and cake shuttling to and fro. But when understaffed, they shift the inmates to the big day room at the front. I have a moment of peace before re-entering the strange and difficult world in which My Love finds herself.

DAY 69, Glasgow, UK

Home is so sad. I have a look at the Larkin poem. It's so quietly desolate, it's funny. After coffee, I hear that Jaine Henderson died last night. As I emerged from My Love's care home around six-thirty yesterday, I contemplated turning left towards the hospital or right for home. I had a long think. Exhaustion got the better of me and I turned right. Exhaustion and moral cowardice. I'm telling myself I'm glad to have my last memory of Jaine sitting up in bed, chatting and laughing. And I can blame the Ghastly Affliction for my lack of courage. The only thing I regret is that I'll never see Jaine again, nor light up when her name lights up my phone.

In the afternoon, I cycle east of town to pick up some guitar strings and cans of G&T for the surviving members of the Henderson clan should they find the gumption to attend the show. So strange that the Dels' and the Minds' mutual friend should die on a day off in Glasgow on this tour.

The bike ride takes me through the area around Glasgow Cross that rings, and rings, and rings with Jaine. That crazy dark bitch, that ladylike friend, that sister of the night. And the light. I stop on the Clyde Walkway by the Kingston Bridge, whose pale concrete suddenly illuminates in a band of sunshine. The vehicles flood inexorably from south to north, north to south. How quickly people slip from light to shade.

DAY 70, Glasgow, UK

There was a short debate between Iain and I last night about how or even if we should acknowledge Jaine's death. Iain decides to play a few bars of Slade's 'Gudbuy T'Jane' and I make the briefest of dedications before the last song. Mawkishness would not have been her thing. But I struggled with emotions for the whole show; Jaine and David and Mary were never off my mind. On occasion, that was beautiful, lending a line new poignancy, but Gavin was out of control, dusting my bass strings between plucks. I hid him behind my back several times in a desperate ploy to prevent him distracting the crowd. Could I wear a sling? Tie him to a rod? Even now he's causing my index finger to hover over every letter with uncertainty. Map manipulation is the worst. You try to zoom out and a spasm causes you to drop a pin. I've dropped more pins on England than the Nazis did bombs in World War II.

The sun is shining through the slats of my studio blinds and I make plans to get up and go to the care home. Luke is sitting on the couch upstairs with girlfriend Bethan, both getting ready to go to work in The Drake, a bar over the hill from the house. It's nice to have young folk around – especially someone I love so dearly who is going through a similar experience dealing with all the guilt and responsibility his mother's incapacity has created. I stop for coffee on the way over the river to see My Love. I find myself in one of those high-ceilinged Victorian shop units with exposed stonework and mismatching second-hand furniture bought in an auction job lot: pot plants and standard lamps, an eager beaver barista, nu-soul on the stereo. It's trying to be funky, but it's a complete dog's breakfast. The coffee is top fucking notch and I decide that I love it. It shall be my new neighbourhood hot beverage haunt.

Bad timing at the care home. My Love is being bathed. Baths were always her thing, though latterly, when she was ailing, she began to fear the water. My Love has a phobia of fountains and both of us always assumed some childhood trauma the cause of this. There are a few family legends involving near-drownings. Some families have fire, some have water.

She emerges like a pampered nymph and is hoisted into bed. I sit for a few hours reading news stories aloud, holding her hand, nuzzling her downy cheek, kissing her red lips. My eyes fill at one point and My Love notices. I lie and say I'm thinking of Jaine.

The show seems less fraught than last night and I swoop into the guest room backstage afterwards still in my gig outfit, like a red-carpet conqueror. There are a few selfies and a lot of what can only be described as subtle sympathy, which I appreciate for what it is – well-meant concern and acknowledgment that WE KNOW, without any drama. I make my excuses after forty minutes and go upstairs to the dressing room to have dinner. Simple Minds' humongous uplift is bouncing around the building. I say goodbye to the security women staffing our corridor and hop on my bike, taking the covered pedestrian overpass spanning the Clydeside Expressway. Buskers pitch up at the two right-angles on this bridge whenever there's a concert. They usually tailor their repertoire to suit the act. The second guy at the far end of the tunnel is playing a guitar so out of tune it sounds like a cat attacking a set of bagpipes. Or maybe the other way around. The Doppler effect as I speed past is pronounced. It's been a strange week. I saw David, Jaine's brother, at our soundcheck. He had that drawn, care-etched skin of the recently bereaved. His hug had worlds in it.

DAY 71, day off, Glasgow, UK

The discrepancy between my watch and phone can only be explained by the commencement of British Summer Time – never as exciting as its title suggests. Spring forward, fall back, grind on. It's also Easter, which I didn't notice until I turned on Radio 4 yesterday and a squall of sanctimoniousness filled the bathroom. Those smug, plaintive hymns – they're vomit-inducing. You know all the singers have spotless pastel outfits and immaculate houses. They're the kind of people who wipe down their vacuum cleaners after every second use.

As the homicide police know, we are creatures of habit, and I return to the same coffee shop on the way to the care home. On ordering a croissant and not yesterday's lemon cake, the barista says, 'Changin' it up!'. I don't know whether to politely ignore this or break down sobbing uncontrollably, flailing at the floor, crying 'Death! Death! Take me! Take me now!'

Her ladyship (as I've noticed some of My Love's friends calling her on her WhatsApp group) is not game this afternoon and I cannot rouse her with gentle coaxing. I decide to sit quietly for a while to see what happens before I scarper. But she stirs and reaches out – not, as you might suspect, for my hand, but to extinguish an imaginary cigarette. My Love must have had a cigarette in her hand or at her side for the majority of her life. Today is not good. She doesn't seem to understand anything I'm saying and her utterances are scatterbrain non-sequiturs. I'm becoming increasingly distressed at what is looking like a long-term trend in her condition. I feel like she's slipping away. I feel like I'm standing at the end of a jetty calling her name into the fog. All that comes back is the dull echo of my own voice.

I cycle home in mild spring air, a glinting sun, the city in a Sunday hush. I speak to Luke about his mother. I'm not sure sharing our concern is helpful. We both want to do something to change her condition but are powerless. It's hopelessness manifesting as bewilderment. I take a walk through the park and sit on a sunny bench, the trees winter bare, a parade of dog walkers passing my perch with their absurdly shaped pooches. A plane takes me out of here tomorrow. I'll leave these losses behind, but they will not lose sight of me.

DAY 72, Glasgow to Luxembourg

Andy picks me up just after midday in a cab. At the check-in, we're offered a cheap upgrade for the London–Luxembourg leg, which I buy for a laugh. It'll give me and Andy something to annoy the others about. It's pathetic, but it has cheered me up. Everything this morning was enervating. I tried to set up the AirTag the Barenaked Ladies team had given us at the end of last year's tour, but my wandering digit had tamped the wrong button and I found myself clumsily fiddling with the tiny disc attempting to force a reboot. I felt like a bear with a pair of tweezers trying to get a splinter out of its paw. The Ghastly Affliction is exasperating some days. One day last month, I couldn't get my dick out of my jeans for a piss. It took me five minutes of maladroit fumbling, like being assaulted by a teenage pervert.

I am seated in an exit row and steward Louise talks us through the evacuation procedure. I study the five illustrations on the back of the seat and realise I don't have a clue what they mean. They could mean:

1. Punch the air
2. Throw a drawing of two sausages on the floor
3. Hang on to the top of the window
4. Tear the window out of the fuselage with the strength of ten men
5. Stay seated and sob into a telescope.

I cheerfully confirm to Louise that I fully understand my respon-
sibilities with the confident smile of a partially deaf simpleton. The
engines strike up that flamethrower sound, joined by various whines
and grinding overhead. I'm sure they're testing the flaps and what-
not, but this pre-take-off racket always sounds like there's a building
site downstairs. The captain is a sickeningly cheerful Englishman who
comes over like a south coast local radio personality. I'd like to smash
his chops in with a big book.

I look down at my horrible clothes, this saggy double-denim uni-
form I've got stuck in for years. It's less Texas Tuxedo, more Man with
No Libido. I'm drab, dad. I would do something about this, but decent
clothes are so impractical. This jaded suit holds so many bits in the
right place – pills over my heart, phone across my liver, wallet on a
kidney. Left arse cheek: mask, right arse cheek: plectrums. Front right:
Leatherman Micra multitool and keys, front left: CASH! It all goes
like clockwork until you mix up stage clobber with street clothes –
because you must never have anything in your pockets on stage you do
not need. On this tour, I have picks and a pass. There's nothing worse
than seeing a clump of change in some performer's pocket. Anyone
who takes a phone on stage is a fake and should be expelled from the
realm of rock.

We touch down and are swallowed by the bowels of Heathrow,
bussed, searched and spat out into the trauma of a packed Terminal 3,
a boiling sea of zombie transfer passengers and glittering rip-off shacks.
It's a horrid place and everybody hates it, but still they sell you sunglasses. At Luxembourg Airport, we quickly find our old driver friend
Simon and his infeasibly big bus in order to be installed in flashy Sofitel
rooms within a few minutes. I break out for a kebab shop through
clean, brightly lit streets, avoiding a congregation of some ten thirty-
year-old men on a narrow side street. I have no idea what they're up

to, but the absence of women makes me nervous. I try to make myself look bigger under my combat coat, but combat is not in my repertoire. I muse how embarrassing it would be to have to tell the tale. 'You were mugged in *Luxembourg*?'

Liberty Kebabs is, like the city, clean and bright, and I mangle some French to get roughly what I desire. A perfectly presentable youngish woman comes up to the window near where I sit and starts convulsing with a profound hacking cough that sounds like it's emanating from a camel. I'm starting to suspect a local opioid problem. People are bedding down in various doorways. Two men meet on a corner and swap indiscernible contraband at crotch height. I walk back past what looks like a castle out in the dark beyond the lamplight. In my room, I flip through every channel once on the huge wall-mounted TV. They speak Luxembourger here, but everything on telly is French or German. The *CIA World Factbook* informs me that the second largest ethnic group is Portuguese, which seems very odd. I can't think of an obvious link. I will ask someone tomorrow. I watch Liam Neeson dubbed into German. As with all German re-voiced films, the timbre and texture is very close to Neeson's whispery Irish growl. I have no idea what he's saying, but I presume he's still running around hitting people while looking for his fucking daughter.

DAY 73, Luxembourg

It's a raw, torn-up day and I suppose you could say the city appears very European – if you wanted to say something meaningless. My room looks on to the Grand Ducal Palace with the conical witch's hat roofs of a Disney castle. But the bus takes us away! Within minutes, we're in countryside. Dammit – this could be a day stuck in the sticks, tolerable when the weather is good but miserable when not. I have a panicky glance at the map. The Rockhal sits on the edge of a university campus in Esch-sur-Alzette, near the French border, at Number 5 Avenue du Rock'n'Roll. I spot the National Museum of the Resistance nearby, so there might be some hope of distraction. I slump in my usual position on a back-lounge bench, watching the gently rolling terrain, shrubs and trees showing the slightest fuzz of colour. We pass the old ArcelorMittal steel plant and enter what looks like an American city in miniature, built last week. From the Greenwich Peninsula in London, I had spotted the ArcelorMittal Orbit through a thicket of hi-rises. It's a disgusting mess of an Anish Kapoor sculpture, erected in 2012 by a dick called Lakshmi Mittal in the London Olympic Park site to celebrate his wealth and status as a steel tycoon. Maybe he built tonight's venue.

I hop off the bus, exit the site and turn into Avenue du Rock'n'Roll to be smacked in the face with the giant plant, a mass of rusting pipes, chimneys and walkways. It's far more impressive than the Kapoor sculpture. An odd-looking German couple approach for an autograph and a photo. 'Are you coming to the show?' I ask. 'No. We are here on our holidays,' the woman replies. I don't think they're fans. They're autograph hounds – those takers of names, collectors of marks, evidence traders, script squirrellers. In the plaza at the venue's front, two men in hi-vis are photographing a group of thin saplings planted into the concrete. Each tree has a collar of fibreglass wool halfway up its trunk, like they're dressed for the opera.

The route to the museum takes me around the edge of town, anticlockwise, industrial yards and transport depots to my left, fields and nondescript terraced houses to my right. It feels like a European rust belt. There are at least ten sets of train tracks between me and the town, the embankment spattered with pale blossom.

The museum is housed in a handsome 1930s building with Speer-esque square columns and Soviet realist-style reliefs set into the frontage. At the reception desk, a woman with long black hair and dark brown eyes earnestly talks me through the exhibits. The building has been renovated very recently and I like it a lot. In the main atrium, each wall has booths with waist-level touchscreens angled like long lecterns. When you highlight a portrait, the person's biography fades up and little physical items are spot-lit on the wall behind. I spend an hour doing this over and over, getting a feel for how the population reacted when the Nazis invaded in 1940.

Everything is in three languages. There's a room upstairs that explores the totalitarianism of the occupiers. I'd forgotten how the National Socialist doctrine was so universally applied. When you think of fascism, you think of the militarism, the belligerence and the absurd fanaticism. But the Third Reich was also driven by crackpot racial theory and pseudo-scientific dogma. Every part of society was Nazified, every oppositional institution destroyed, from monasteries to political parties, sports clubs to art societies. The indoctrination was total, obsessive and brutal. It's a very successful museum, imparting information and deepening one's knowledge in a clear, concise and seductive way.

I stroll about the quaint town for a while, peering through the tinted windows of unwelcoming cafés before I decide to head back. It's a weird mixture of the smug and faintly sordid. I walk through the swanky railway station, which resembles a silver slug. I scoff two bowls of soup and a cream horn in a pleasant catering room three storeys up in the big concrete box of the Rockhal. I do not feel at all ready to rock this hal. Then I remember I've missed a pill.

I go into a bit of a mood coma pre-gig, but the meds kick in on time and the adrenaline makes me laugh. I think most of the audience like us but it's hard to tell. They're not very demonstrative, nor seem to be later when I watch the Minds from the back of the floor. I feel like Jim Kerr is struggling to feel anything coming back from them. I go outside and sit on a bench in the plaza in front of the venue. The big, heavy chords of 'Belfast Child' swim out into the damp evening air. A couple say hi. 'You were very good.'

I always wanted my gravestone to read:

'I Wasn't That Good'

DAY 74, day off, Strasbourg, France

I am gently shaken awake in my bunk by Derek around 11 a.m. I have on my noise cancellers, so physical contact is necessary. He has a father's careful touch and I'm grateful for it. I dozily pack my shit and get off pronto, aware of the bus's imminent disappearance to somewhere on the periphery. It's a block or two to the Sofitel and I'm in room 209 and unpacking for ten minutes when I realise I've left my phone in my bunk. I quickly check my back pocket for my room key and race down the three flights of stairs, run through a little square to the main drag, turn right and... the bus is still there. Iain is getting his fold-up bike out of the bay. Thank fuck. I thank Simon and we chat about thinking your phone's missing when you're actually holding it. This sickness. I'd already considered that it would have been so inconvenient to get the thing back today that the best plan would be to remain phoneless 'til midday tomorrow, a scenario I was already looking forward to. I could have bought a little notebook for my thoughts and used the map the hotel had issued me to navigate.

I establish that I am on an island in the River Ill called Grande Île and therefore located in the historic centre. I punch in the Gallery of

Modern Art to discover it closes between 1 and 2 p.m. How can that ever be worth it? Closing between twelve and three I could understand. At the stroke of midday, an air-raid siren sounds, followed by much ringing of church bells. I have no idea why. So, I look it up. It's a 'reminder' siren and has been sounding for a minute in every French town since World War II on the first Wednesday of each month. That I don't know this shows how little time I've spent in the country. In a survey quoted in the article, 78 per cent of people would do nothing if the real siren went off. So, really, it's just a 'fuck you' to the Germans. Fuck you, you know you want to. Mneeeaaawwwwwww!

I put on Neil Young's *On the Beach* and snooze until three. I meet Iain at the front door getting his bike unfolded. I think he's hungover, but you'd be hard pushed ever to get him to admit to such a thing. I look into a church ten metres from the hotel. It has red sandstone pillars and peeling frescoes. There's a gaudy organ whose pipes reach up to the vaulted roof in a frame of gold and salmon pink. It's freezing and damp, but I notice some beautiful stained glass in the nave which I have to crane my neck to see. The blues and reds are as sharp as an acid trip. There's a very dark oil painting of a crucified Jesus above the door. Only the body is discernible, and the absence of a cross makes it look like the figure is doing a big happy dance. If he was saying anything, it would be 'Whoopee!'. I stick a fiver in a slotted box and get back to the relative warmth of the outdoors.

The first thing that strikes me is that this is one quiet town. There is very little traffic, perhaps because there are a lot of trams. I flounce up a shopping street (it could be Munich), cross the narrow river at a weir, hang left and I'm at the Musée d'Arte Moderne, featuring a fabulous long high atrium with flying walkways amid much glass panelling. In the forecourt, I admire a just-larger-than-life-size bronze man who looks like he's been squeezed out of a piping bag, like a cross between the Michelin Man and Mr Whippy. His hands end in a creamy peak and I feel sorry for him, despite his jaunty stride. Maybe he's drunk or maybe he's desperate. His mouth is hidden under one of the whirls of his face, held in a distorted 'O' of sharp pain. I note later it's by Thomas Schütte and made in the late '90s. Everything is nicely mixed up – Impressionism, Surrealism, Cubism and 21st-century ephemera. I can't say I'm ever bored.

There's a pair of classic black and grey Picassos from the mid-1920s, the larger of which, *Femme à la guitare*, looks like he tossed it off in fifteen minutes. There's a crappy Magritte with a volcano made out of white hair and some idealised tits. I really like a tall bronze by Markus Lüpertz called *Hirte* (Shepherd) from 1986. He's grey and skinny with a big red face, like he's been on the Special Brew in the park all day. He has a lamb draped over his shoulders, except it can't be a lamb because it has horns. It reminds me of the story of my father's about finding a lost lamb while walking high up in the hills and descending with it in his rucksack. He found a single ewe lower on the mountain, but she wasn't interested. He carried the lamb down to the road and found the shepherd who said, 'I wondered where that'd gone'.

The grey figure is planted beside an enormous hulk of a plaster Rodin penseur and I know who's won this particular face-off. There's some gimmicky pointillist stuff (a hideous Signac landscape in pink and lime green) and a cavernous roomful of Gustave Doré Passion scenes, one of which is bigger than my house. Here are my three sents: sensationalist, sentimental and sententious. They are also laughably histrionic. Jesus looks like a Vegas magician levitating down the Via Dolorosa as if lit by a mirrorball. Upstairs, I find what I recognise as Angry Richard Ashcroft but is captioned 'Jonathan Meese, *Selbst als Kapitain Danjou*', a self-portrait by a German artist from 2000. I also spot a very good Max Ernst called *À l'intérieur de la vue*, an enchanting jumble of tussling birds framed in an ellipse. I love the building. It is beautiful and refined, simple to understand, easy to use.

I meander onto the Barrage Vauban, a seventeenth-century covered bridge with a pathway on its roof looking on to a delightful medieval river scene. I pass a curious thing – a cruddy column of disintegrating render climbing up a new building. At first, I think it must be an art piece until I glean it's one of those living walls gone bad. All the mosses and ferns have died, leaving gaping slits of dead brown compost trailing down. It's kind of cool. I look up and two cyclists crash into each other. Words are said, jackets dusted down. They look flustered, but part before the blaming starts. I blame the cycle paths which are too narrow. I'd use the road. But then you have the tram tracks. Satisfyingly, I later pass a man, the spitting image of Ian McKellen, wearing a beret and fawn raincoat. After a cheap pizza, I stroll through the narrow streets of the old town, all watch shops and boulangeries. The cathedral is red and grotesquely ornamented, covered in saints and deer and gargoyles. I pass a shop that sells globes and pens; another sells shoe polish, laces and zips. The centre is very quiet, very rich. It's not unlike York in its layout. I walk back to my big bed and sleep to the sweet twang of early Lynyrd Skynyrd. Perhaps the Yanks should broadcast 'Freebird' across America every month to show Putin they're good and ready. I can't say I love Strasbourg. It's like Brad Pitt. Wealthy, good looking and a bit dull.

DAY 75, Strasbourg, France

We drive over the Canal du Faux-Rempart, which serves as a city moat. Two tooled-up soldiers cross in front of the bus, sleek and menacing in berets and camouflage with both hands on their assault weapons.

The way they're looking around and working as a team looks more like an operation than a routine patrol. I never feel safer in the presence of automatic weapons. From a motorway flyover, I see a shanty town of makeshift huts and mud-clogged streets wedged in a sliver of land between slip roads. There's rubbish strewn around, cinder blocks holding down plastic tarpaulins. The last time I saw such a thing was Portugal in the mid-'80s. A military cemetery, manicured and immaculate, sits just beyond the camp, the dead having better conditions than the living. We pull into a soulless industrial estate, turn a few corners until the enormous salmon pink structure of the Zenith appears like an alien spaceship modelled on a blancmange. It looks like the dimension from which yesterday's Mr Whippy came. It looks like a pile of taramasalata.

I fuel up in catering; me, Andy, Kris and Jim at one table, four bus drivers at another. I hear the band's tales of last night's manoeuvres, a few of them spotting an interesting-looking bar only to discover it was a brothel. 'We thought it a bit odd that we had to get buzzed in.' I leave my bag in a dismal dressing room and make a beeline for a shopping centre in the absence of any better options in the area. I drift in, I drift out. I stand in the sock aisle. I parade past the Bluetooth speakers. I study some teabags. At a junction outside, I watch two men unroll cable from a drum and thread it through a manhole. The air has an Atlantic smell and there's a hint of heat in it. Strasbourg has exported its noise to these outskirts. There's a bland wall of mechanical noise all around. I'm as bored as a brat.

I notice on the map that all the towns on the French side along the Rhine have Germanic names, but there are no Francophone names on the German side. The stupidity of borders. Back at catering, I cast my eyes over a collage of black and white artist portraits hung on a long wall. I do not recognise any of them. A woman I assume to be Sharleen

Spiteri turns out on closer inspection to be no one of the sort. Finally, I find Seal and just below him a little Elton in that familiar hunch-shouldered pose at the piano. One of the caterers is singing 'Don't You Forget About Me'. Her colleague sticks on some Travis to drown her out. The song is 'Sing'. Hey Fran! Sing that Sing hing!

Somebody asked me recently if there is a recognisable strain that runs through Scottish pop music. I think there is. I can't quite put my finger on it, but there's a melodic connection between the Fire Engines and Boards of Canada, a strange kinship between Young Fathers and the Blue Nile. I can hear a new song on radio and know it's Scottish. Our 'ooh's are tight, our 'ee's have an edge. It's a sensibility, not a style.

I have a miraculously enjoyable gig. One show out of ten is so easy, so much joy. Some days, the disease decides to take a day off. I make fewer gaffes than usual, my voice does what I ask of it and some of my bass playing is tight. I ruefully regard the uninterested few hundred dotted about the place: *You don't understand – this is good!* The house lights go up and down during our set, so I can see the blank faces. I remain a star in my own mind.

DAY 76, Antwerp, Belgium

I wake up on the stroke of midday feeling well. In catering, Andy and Iain, having already been out and about, give me the lowdown. The metro sounds the best bet. I circumnavigate the arena to get to the underground, taking an escalator into a large ticket foyer and quickly getting orientated. Piece of piss. I travel from Sport to Opera, which keeps things simple. On my phone, I plug in a museum address and follow the blue line, stumbling across an English-language bookshop en route. I buy four slim Penguins that should fill the void left by finishing Jim Thompson's *Pop. 1280* last night. What a sordid book. I felt sullied reading it. Incest, faithlessness and psychopathy with some well-written sex thrown in. Recommended.

The sun burns through the murk and I sit on a wooden bench in Leopoldplaats, the man himself heroically astride a snorting charger on a high granite plinth. I'm judging by the date on the statue that this fellow is not the Cunt of the Congo but one of his forebears. Some quick checking confirms him as the Cunt's dad, King Leopold the First. Number two was the unspeakable coloniser of the Congo, the Rubber King – slaver, torturer, amputator. I don't imagine there are many effigies of him left around town. That cunt got cancelled in the nineteenth century.

Antwerp is charming. Cobblestones, trams and chocolate-box buildings. It's a little Amsterdammy, but not as ridiculously pretty; a bit more functional and stately. The narrow streets lead through a series of circular seven-street junctions and open out onto a grand square, the imposing facade of the KMSKA, the Royal Museum of Fine Arts, looming over me like a neoclassical super-tanker. I buy a ticket for €20 from a touchscreen dispenser and slip through the crowds of bovine rubbernecks and take as quick a tour as I can. They have ingeniously brought daylight into every floor of the gallery, creating an ambient wash over everything. Sadly, I can't find anything that hooks. There's a ton of Rik Wouters from the late nineteenth and early twentieth centuries, but it looks highly derivative to me. I enjoy Pieter Brueghel II's *The People's Census at Bethlehem*: the busy little people, the crows sitting in judgement high up on skeletal branches etched against a winter sky.

Downstairs, in a dimly lit case, are two lovely Rodins – a head of Rose Beuret and a depiction of Polyphemus, an exquisitely hewn thing about the size of a human hand. I walk through the dark blue rooms of the paper exhibits, all Rubens-related etchings, and take a steep marble staircase down into a sunken gallery with a high ceiling where I am greeted by a purring translucent fibreglass cat in an open cage. It is glowing from within with aurora-style moving lighting, has one red and one green eye and occasionally emits high-pitched 'Allo's and 'Bonjour's along with its relentless purr. I can't get enough of it. It's so funny. It's sitting there facing a wall of enormous monstrosities by James Ensor, some faux Impressionist from the late 1800s. It's openly mocking them. I can find no information on this sarcastic pussy, a QR code on the floor taking me to a page of impenetrable Flemish. I'd happily have it in my house. Allo! Bonjour!

I'm running short of time and, realising I've missed out the whole Old Masters wing, decide to do a lightning tour. I swan past a famous Brueghel I, leave a roomful of huge gory Christs in my wake to be stopped by a tiny *Give the People What They Want* by Marlene Dumas, a young girl holding open her bath towel with an inscrutable look. It's the antidote to all those nineteenth-century idealised prepubescent girls depicted by sleazy men. On the way out, side by side are Jan Brueghel I's marvellous *The Tower of Babel* and a magnificent Dalí – *Landscape with Girl Skipping Rope*. Both paintings are vast canvases, and both use scale brilliantly.

I grab my sack from locker 39, punching in my universal four-digit PIN. You get that number, you get everything. There appear to be no metro stations near, so I get hiking on the long straight line of Nationalestraat. The city is magnificent in the warm spring sunshine. I squeeze onto my train, straphanging until a seat becomes vacant. How amazing human beings are at pretending to ignore one another. I'm practically sitting in these people's laps, yet not a jot of acknowledgment passes between us. But we're all casting sly glances over one another when we think we won't be noticed. I get back to the

Sportpaleis bang on time to have coffee and cake before soundcheck in its black, cavernous void.

I watch a couple of songs of Simple Minds' set from stage left. They make such a massive, awesome racket. I look around the crowd, stacked way up into the high roof, faces lit by the dazzling light spilling from the stage. They're in a state of wonder.

It's a balmy evening. I imagine people in town sitting in squares, smoking and drinking. I imagine My Love lying in bed waiting for another day of hell to begin. The bitter sap of guilt rises through me. I tell myself to enjoy this for what it is – a long farewell. Moments of joy among the murderous diminishing.

DAY 77, Amsterdam, Netherlands

A bunk map check at 11.30 a.m. reveals what I feared. The venue is more than an hour from the city on foot. Google throws up a reachable modern art place, OSCAM, the Open Space Contemporary Art Museum. The pictures look a delight. I have trouble following the mad loop of a route and figure the map is trying to take me on a wild goose chase to access a pedestrian flyover when I can just make a dash across the highway right here. I'm suddenly doing a circuit of the Johan Cruyff Arena, Ajax's amazing hi-tech football ground. It stands like a sci-fi castle surrounded by a filthy moat, roads flying into its armoured sides.

The sun is out and I ditch the hoodie for the first time this tour. The breeze is high but carries the moist warmth of the ocean. I walk under the huge futuristic train station into a brick-paved plaza – everything clean and bright and new – and on to a newly built retail/residential zone, beautifully proportioned and immaculately laid out. It looks like the architect's idealised drawing of some 1970s English satellite town pedestrian shopping centre, those wind-tunnel hellscapes that blight many places in the UK. But they've got this so right: five-storey apartments over high-ceilinged shop units, pleasant squares with mature trees. No cars, just birdsong and the low mumble of people going about their business in a built environment that considered them first in its design. I don't miss the city at all. I have coffee outside and watch the chill Dutch mingle. There's an old yellow ambulance with an awning attached reading 'Jezus roept ook jou!' The rear doors say, 'Soul Rescue'. But the evangelists themselves are sitting quietly on deckchairs, annoying nobody. Later on, they meekly hand out leaflets almost apologetically. That's my kind of promo.

The gallery is a small two-room space. The current show is a celebration of Amsterdam's hip-hop bar, Café De Duivel. Flyers, graffiti, video screens, a mock-up of the bar. It gives me a pretty good idea of what the place was like in the '90s and zeroes. I ponder whether Glasgow ever had a hip-hop bar. I'm not sure Glasgow ever had a hip bar.

I dip into a TK Maxx out of sheer boredom, immediately feel trapped and make a sharp exit. There's a 'second-hand' clothes shop on a corner which, like all these purportedly vintage outlets, is full of rubbish, mostly never worn. Real stuff from the '70s and before moved online years ago. And all my '70s suits that I sported in the late zeroes have suffered death by moth, the crotch-munching bastards.

I have a repulsive omelette baguette on the terrace of a huge, deserted restaurant, the sun now beating from a high angle. I'm bathing in it. The waiter stands in the doorway three feet away while I eat, making me feel he thinks I'm a flight risk. A trumpet is playing somewhere. There's not a combustion engine to be heard anywhere in the vicinity. People of every social class and ethnicity stroll, cycle and scooter around. It looks like the European dream of the integrated, prosperous, open society. And if it looks like that, there's a chance it might be that. Across the square, I see a waitress sail into a forest of tables holding aloft a tray of three foaming beers. I feel the sun's rays stretching my shallow skin. I live a little in that easy minute.

I watch fifteen minutes of the latter part of the Minds set, the audience agog, the stage lights splashing about the three cliffs of faces, glowing from without and within. The big, big noise. The communal climax. As Mr Kerr says, satisfied customers. I sit at the top of a fire escape staircase waiting for Simon to wake up and fix the heating on our freezing bus. Cars crawl on a bridge above, on the road below. Reuben the stage manager has some ribs delivered to our bus from a local barbecue place he knows. I wolf delicious lamb and pork atavistically. It's been so long since I ate real meat, my body goes into a kind of reverie – a flesh fever. Finally, we get on the road around midnight. I have Joni Mitchell's *The Hissing of Summer Lawns* up real loud. The Netherlands gets left in our slipstream. I'm sad to see them go.

DAY 78, day off, Copenhagen, Denmark

I get into my nineteenth-floor cell at midday. Copenhagen is laid before me; steep, red-tiled roofs and copper-topped spires, turbines revolving out on the coast, a warship in dock. I take a pedestrian bridge over the Stadsgraven canal into a park; swans sailing serenely, Sunday strollers, canine carers, puffed-out joggers. The sun is singeing the clouds just enough to warm the skin. I see a message from Brian that he's in The Dubliner watching the Celtic game. For want of any other inspiration, I set controls for there, imagining it to be too busy to tolerate on a day off. I follow the blue dotted line through cobbled lanes to a square hosting a small convention for young alcoholics. They have a plastic crate of beer in brown bottles. They have luggage in a pile and some are having trouble remaining vertical. A few hundred metres on, I am tempted into a canal-side café for breakfast. It's an organic, seed-obsessed place, but the food turns out to be brilliant. My multi-juice comes with a steel straw which immediately makes me think of cocaine. What do I know of cocaine? Not much. Except that it's only effective at levels of purity rarely found in Europe, when the come-down is merciless and you're left contemplating the murder, poverty and corruption you have helped perpetuate. Apart from that, knock yourself out. Of course, it should be legally obtainable and licensed like alcohol.

The Dubliner proves to be not too rammed and I'm greeted by two of the Minds crew at the door who direct me to Brian. 'Yer man's in a green jumper.' Naturally. We watch a pretty terrible second-half Celtic performance, the two of us muttering and shaking our heads. There's the usual pointless shouting and swearing at every decision that goes Rangers' way. There's plenty of drama, a VAR reversal with a penalty given and an open-play goal taken away by the same process. Celtic score to make it 2–3 in the final minutes, only for Rangers to equalise in time added on. The young Irish couple at our table seem happy with a draw, Brian and I less so. But, in the end, it's bread and circuses. None of it matters, and all of it distracts.

I'm spat out into the daylight, 0.5 per cent beer swilling around my belly like a trailing anchor. I get sucked into the same shopping streets as two years ago. I need a loo and things to do. I need an art museum. But I'm running out of time and decide to float. Let's see where my nose goes. I meander through a delightful little cobbled square to the Christiansborg Palace, taking a bench under a tree and gazing at the shimmering water in the canal. The bird above me is marking its territory with an irritatingly repetitive three-note sequence, two high, one a fifth lower. I've heard more melodic burglar alarms. Tourist boats sail by under the low, ornate bridge of Marmorboden and I strain to catch some morsel of information from the tour guides. Most of the rental boats have electric outboard motors and slip through the water with a mere purr. The boring bird finally fucks off and I feel it is time I did the same.

Back at the penthouse, I recline in my easy chair and watch the lowering sunlight pick out Copenhagen's greens and russets. I'm reading Camus' *Reflections on the Guillotine* and nodding off. I come to at eight, wisps of pink cloud hanging in a sky of electric blue. Outside the hotel, I walk away from the city through a new upmarket housing estate to a café that has stopped serving food earlier than advertised. As I slouch back disconsolately, I spy a very welcoming-looking establishment called Il Buco, which I assume is a neighbourhood Italian. But as I'm led to a table opposite the open kitchen, I figure different. Oh – a tasting menu… Still, I'm here now, fuck it. Bring me five courses! Bring me the finest produce of Denmark! Sod the proletariat – this is dinner with the bourgeoisie. I order two oysters to start, which come beautifully presented on a little plate of bleached shells among which hides a pipette for applying a lemongrass vinaigrette. Then a fizzy, sweet amuse-bouche (with ice cube and purple flowers) heralds a board of charcuterie – a rough pâté, some cured pork and a meatloaf – all deliciously salty and perfectly accompanied by some spicy fermented aubergine. Hot on its heels is mushroom toast, earthy and meaty, topped with a dusting of Gruyère. Next is a nest of chunky homemade pasta in a herby sea-green paste, followed by a bloody chunk of duck the size of an eclair. This duck sure had big tits. It's exquisitely seasoned with a subtle sauce and some buttery leek and endive garnish. It's all just the right side of poncey and too delicious to carp about. Plus, it's washed down with two bottles of Don't Worry, a locally sourced IPA and by far the best zero-alcohol beer I've tasted. The waitress tries to sell me a cheese course before dessert, but I'm not falling for it. I'm Monsieur Creosote here, baby. Ready to blow! The dessert – preceded by an incredible apple-scented palate-cleanser sorbet on a frozen spoon – is simply mind-blowing. A localised version of tiramisu, the base is soaked in more alcohol than has passed my lips since before Christmas. This has been my *Babette's Feast*.

As I'm dabbing my lips with my small square of textured cotton, I think of how My Love is so fastidious when she eats, constantly reaching for a napkin to wipe around her mouth. It's a sad and delicate action, and the thought of it leaves me feeling the same. My stomach is full of rich, fine fare. My heart is empty of all desire other than to go back, back to before all this shit began. She would have loved this food, and we would have had wine, and smoked cigarettes on the way home, laughing in the cooling night.

DAY 79, Copenhagen, Denmark

I load my luggage onto the bus, fill my bottle and jump off. I'm going to do a bit more exploring before hitting the arena, which is out of town. I head for Home of Carlsberg. My friend Damien's company ISO, who designed my four solo sleeves, did the installation for the museum here and I told him I'd take a look. It's an hour's hike west along the quayside which, like Belfast and Dublin, has been extensively redeveloped. I can't see a single thing not built in the last twenty years. It's springtime again today and the walking is easy. I enter the old Carlsberg brewery complex and buy a ticket from a machine (although human beings are available). It looks very like the Highland Park whisky distillery we visited three years ago, various brick outhouses linked by cobbled streets, a chimney or two. I have to wait in a doorway for ten minutes until my timeslot, whereupon two young Danes with strap-on smiles usher the six of us who've gathered into a theatrically lit warehouse room furnished with a large square bar. Small glasses of beer are handed out and there's a preamble before we're mercifully left to our own devices.

The tour starts upstairs with long video screens depicting supersimple, bite-sized chunks of the brewery's dull history. There's some nice lighting and the 3D-animated story snippets remind me of Ladybird books. Some of the company mottos are written in suspended type on wires, all in gold and dramatically illuminated from above. Everything is company propaganda. For example, there is no video content illustrating the role of Carlsberg Special Brew in the development of the Great British derelict. I am less than fascinated to learn that the brand was named after the original brewer's son, Carl, who went on to piss his dad off something rotten by compromising the quality of the product to expand and produce higher volumes. So, absurdly, there was New Carlsberg and Old Carlsberg in direct competition for a period. I'm losing the will to live as I absorb this. How interesting can the history of a brewery be? Okay, they used the ancient symbol of the swastika as a logo for a bit and ditched it when the Nazis co-opted it. Jesus, is that *it*? I'm beginning to regret not taking one of the lagers offered in the foyer bar.

Further on, there's an impressive wall of video screens that you activate by standing under a spotlight and a fabulous cellar room of floor-to-ceiling glass cases holding the thousands of different bottled products the company has issued. It's like Damien Hirst's *Pharmacy* bar for dipsomaniacs. After an hour, I've had enough and speed-walk through the old machinery and mock-up of the Liverpool FC boot room to the exit where I pass through a vast deserted bar to find myself in some stables, reeking richly of manure with a few bronze-coloured dray horses in stalls munching on feed. I wait to be served in the restaurant, but it's a slow Monday and no one's bothered, so I start walking the hour and a half to the venue. The first section is leafy Hampstead-style suburbia, giving way at the bottom of the hill to lower-income neighbourhoods, primary schools, flats with little balconies and a small colony of drunks in a corner park imbibing the very brew invented by J.C. Jacobsen about which I have just been so enlightened.

The route looks like a slog, so I nip in to a Lebanese café on the way to steel my resolve. The barista has her phone tucked into her head scarf so that it's wedged against her cheek. I compliment her on her ergonomic inventiveness. My flatbread is a hearty chickpea and spinach affair, the coffee good and pungent with a medical tinge. I march on alongside a busy ring road, before crossing under several motorways until I find myself in a semi-rural edgeland passing a pistol shooting range, shots eerily ringing out all about me like I've stumbled upon an assassins' training camp. Part of it is laid out like an adventure playground, so grown men can play 'army', 'cowboy' or 'secret spy mission'. On the other side of the path, a flock of geese stand about on the shore of a small lake looking concerned. In the distance, I can see the lettering of the Royal Arena. It looks like a casino. Of course, as is par for the course, there's a golf course. Sadly, none of the putting tits are out today, leaving me unable to get a good loathing on. Perhaps one day there will be war between the pistol people and the golf men, all desperately trying to get their projectiles into one another's holes.

The final stretch has me doglegging through a lovely housing estate, big windows, high- and low-rise brick-faced buildings, staggered to form welcoming courtyards and pretty alleyways, not at all unlike the old Carlsberg brewery. They can design, the Danes. Perhaps it helps that it's all so flat. Every now and then, among the placid pedal-pushing mums and laid-back electric-bike dads, you spot a hard bastard – face like rock and hair like fire – and you remember. They're Vikings.

DAY 80, day off, Hamburg, Germany

Derek wakes me with a soothing urgency. The bus is five minutes from the hotel but can't stop there. Battle stations. Pack USB to lightning cable. Check. Pack USB-3 cable. Check. Pack laundry. Check. Pack toilet bag. Check. Pack headphones. Check. Check weather. Check.

The Tortue Hotel is boutique. We're greeted by two dapper blokes in hot blue suits, white sneakers and carefully tended facial hair. The rooms have 16-foot-high ceilings, two toilets, kitchen, lounge and separate bedroom. I have a shower, a bath, three sinks and a dishwasher. There is a fresh flower arrangement on a half-moon table. The place looks like it was painted yesterday. It's absurd, living in these little oases of luxury when my own house is such a hovel – sheets and towels piled up, books in a great landslide from inadequate shelving, filth, squalor and, in some crevices, twenty years of dust. Even the cat must consider it a bit shoddy, and she sleeps outside in a bush.

I set a course to some kunst, but have trouble motivating myself. Should I nap? I put some music on. Zzzz. I wake at half-two with something very interesting playing – Mount Kimbie and King Krule's 'Empty and Silent'. Great lyrics. So, up I get and head for the Museum für Kunst und Gewerbe. I'm pretty art-ed out by this point, but I obediently trudge through spitting rain and a festering wind to get my daily dose of kultur. The collection of decorative arts and design is housed in a purpose-built three-storey lump opened in 1877. There's a shit ton of between-the-wars deco that feels a bit too familiar, but there is some beautiful glassware, and the recreated rooms are quite magical. I pass two brilliant posters by Annik Troxler, a forty-five-year-old Swiss graphic artist. On the mezzanine, I walk through a large collection of early keyboard instruments – spinets, clavichords and harpsichords – every one accompanied by a Do Not Touch notice. I'm desperate to hear just one pluck. We had a harpsichord in the hall of the third house I grew up in. Tricky things to get a tune out of when you can't play. Pianos, with their sustain pedals, are much easier for beginners. A house without a piano is an impoverished place.

Back outside, I stand on the stone steps watching a stream of dissolute people wandering into an inebriated crowd forming on the far side of the plaza. I try to work out what's going on and can only come up with Festival of the Fucked. I weave back through central Hamburg's stately streets, crossing bridges, squares and courtyards. People check you out here like we do in Glasgow. But at home it is, firstly, to confirm the stranger is not a threat and, secondly, to make sure it's not someone you know. Here, it seems more like disdainful curiosity, as if people are mildly disgusted by their own morbid interest.

I warm myself in the private palace of my room before venturing in the opposite direction from today's barren expedition, coming upon a neighbourly square at the top of a hill. In Paulaner's, I order schnitzel and a quenching zero weisbier. I've been feeling out of sorts since speaking on the phone to Luke in the morning. That conversation has taken me out of touring world and put me back in the world of care and strife. I tried to not let it affect me, but I've been unsettled. I remind myself that there's nothing to be done until I return. Even then, there is little to be done but live in the pain and anguish of watching a lover trapped in an inescapable hell.

DAY 81, Hamburg, Germany

I decide to board the bus bound for the out-of-town venue rather than spending another day walking and worrying about getting to soundcheck on time. The Barclays Arena sits beside the Hamburger SV football stadium north-west of the city. I take an amble through

Volkspark, an uninteresting trek on a paved road through thin forest. It's cooler today and I'm back in the combat jacket. I head for a memorial on the other side of some open parkland where two gentlemen are throwing a series of frisbees exceptional distances. They look like they're training for something. They walk the 150 metres or so and collect their missiles. One has a little caddy over his shoulder to keep them in. They begin throwing again. The older and fatter of the two (wearing a flat cap) is the superior competitor. He throws from shoulder height and releases the frisbee with such a snap that it speeds out of his grip startlingly quickly. His throws gain more height and achieve greater distances than his colleague's, who launches lower and more slowly, sometimes catching a thermal that give his discs surprising length. The things are in the air for as much as five seconds. A third man with a shoulder caddy joins them and commences warm-up throws. It's all beginning to get ridiculous. I move on.

The path takes me through a gate into a circular park, planted around a central 20-foot-high steel cross that's surrounded by a ring of ghoulish weeping willows. Everywhere I look there are gravestones and memorial slabs. I don't know what this is – a graveyard or a garden. I sit on a slatted bench and hot sunshine breaks through. I'm sunbathing among the dead. Through bushes, I see a woman cleaning a headstone. An aphid lands on my jacket and I draw it onto my finger for a closer look until it flies away. Two big bumblebees are pollinating yellow flowers over my shoulder. A helicopter scrapes the canopy of cloud overhead. I can hear a power tool grinding somewhere. The distinctive nee-naw of a European police siren, crows cawing, the cheeping of smaller birds. A grandmother trundles a pram around the circuit. I say hello when she reaches me and she looks through me like I'm nothing.

I read some of the stones. There are no epitaphs, just names, birth and death dates. I see two wives who made it into their nineties, surviving their husbands by thirty years or more. The husbands, born at the dawn of the twentieth century, died in the '60s in their sixties before coronary medicine caught up and evened up the odds between the sexes. There are Viktors and Helgas, Hermans and Ottos.

On the road by the arena, I spot a sleek black structure at the junction. Assuming it to be a shopping centre, my phone reveals it to be the Montblanc pen museum. Bring it on! I enter through the café and find a snooty man at a long desk in a pristine, cream-coloured foyer who sells me a €14 ticket. This takes the form of a cardboard tag upon which I am encouraged to write my name using one of the company's famous fountain pens. I have to hand it to them – the fucker writes as smoothly as a brush with nary a splotch. The museum is to be found at the top of a sweeping curved staircase, the type you might find in a Fred Astaire movie.

The first item for consideration is a circular screen, inside of which one is encouraged to sit. All that seems to happen is the word 'write' floats about in fifty languages. There's not even any music. This hugely disappointing start is swiftly augmented by text boards composed of the sort of pretentious corporate newspeak that gives public relations a bad name. There are jet-black display cases featuring, well, an awful lot of pens. There are pictures of famous people signing important-looking documents with Montblanc pens. Gorbachev! Obama! John F Kennedy! The Queen! There are old pens and less old pens. There are old adverts for pens. In the second room – yes, there's more – there are nibs, more pens, some machine tools and more pens. There are video screens showing pen videos, there is a case full of old ink bottles, and five little display windows, beautifully lit it must be said, featuring pen tops. The accompanying text continues the company gibberish. 'For an artist, everything can be a canvas.' That's about decorative pen lids. It could be about a serial killer.

There's no one around. I start to feel like I'm in a luxury goods shop in an airport where all the other passengers have been drugged and dragged away. There's a big white table laid out with leather-bound writing pads and pens. You take a stool, hook the pen up to a tablet and whatever you draw on the paper comes up on a tablet embedded in the desk beside you. It's a neat trick. The marks visitors have made appear on a video wall, superimposed over one another so they resemble a black smoke of scribble. I wait for a while for my little line drawing to come up. It appears to have been rejected.

After a final room of underwhelming artwork commissions, I descend a second set of marble stairs, my leather soles clicking as if in anticipation of an imminent outburst of tap dancing. Everything is white like cartridge paper. Naturally, the ausgang leads me through the geschenkeladen. I walk the gauntlet, conspicuously ignoring the goods on display, but can't help noticing leather headphones and handbags. Oh, and some pens.

The show is tricky for me. I can't get into it at all. I just grit my teeth and try to get it done. But the last three of four have been enjoyable, despite my shortcomings, so I let this one go. I watch a bit of a Champions League game on Brian's Kindle, but tiredness hits me like a slide tackle and I retire to the bus.

DAY 82, Berlin, Germany

I am asleep early and wake around nine, wondering where I might be. I suspect Cologne and am pleasantly surprised to discover we are parked in the middle of Berlin. I punch in frühstück and I'm off, over the River Spree into Kreuzberg and breakfast outside under trees in new leaf. There are little plots of garden between the road and the pavement, Café Casero's patch featuring iron baths planted with roses.

With the elevated train track, broad streets and warm sunshine, it's all very Brooklyn, if less insufferably hip. I do a bit of research, but can't turn up an interesting destination. The Ramones Museum is half an hour's walk away but looks insubstantial. Besides, I saw the Ramones in 1979 and Joey's little pot belly lives on in the museum of my mind.

I meander. I find a lovely church, St Kate's, set back from the street and hidden behind a statue, and peer through the gates into its plain interior. A crucified Jesus hangs from the roof without a safety net. Around the corner, I spend an hour rifling through the racks of Trendy Army Store, which very much offers what it promises on the sign above the door. I buy socks and some shorts. It's nice to buy everything in pairs. I loop back around to the river and contemplate visiting the Wall Museum. From across the Spree, someone starts to strum an electric guitar. The voice is throaty and thin, a bit Jaggeresque. Willows trail their fingers in the water. The busker goes from 'Stand by Your Man' to Aztec Camera's 'Oblivious'.

The Wall Museum is at the top of two flights of narrow stairs in a dilapidated-looking building on the eastern side. An avuncular chap with big round glasses and a handlebar moustache happily accepts my cash and ushers me into a tiny screening room. I've seen all this before. The various rooms are crammed with mannequins dressed in East German border guard uniforms, holding machine guns just to ram home who the bad guys are here. There are the obligatory video screens everywhere. There's a bit of railway track with an old pram between the rails. It's all a bit claustrophobic and cheap, so an enormous improvement on yesterday's antiseptic opulence. In the room depicting the fall, Richard Strauss's *Also Sprach Zarathustra* is ringing out. It's supposed to be a hallelujah moment, but it's a bit tawdry. And very stuffy.

After that, to my horror, is a little room dedicated to Pink Floyd with footage of a be-mulleted Roger Waters honking out his turgid whine at Potsdamer Platz in 1990. I am keen to gain some air and steer through the last two rooms sharpish. Outside, there's a section of the wall, about 15-foot high with an overhanging rounded top making any clambering tricky. The physical barrier itself isn't terribly daunting. You've got to reckon, with a decent plan involving a ladder, a trampoline and some shoe polish, this thing is surmountable. It's the fuckers with the guns that'd put you right off. Would you risk your life for democratic freedoms? Right now? Or would you hedge your bets, knuckle down and put up with the queues, the austerity, the arbitrary arrests, the restrictions of liberty? I'm not risking death for a cappuccino, although I might for a Ramones' album. *Rocket to Russia* is my favourite.

Back at the Uber Arena, I watch the Minds' soundcheck. Mr Kerr is in the stalls conducting the band through a new number. He's the consummate bandleader, encouraging and pushing the musicians, walking around the auditorium, listening to them play without him. He sits in the first row of the bleachers, hands behind his head, raising them in praise when Sarah Brown sings. The other self-described non-musician he calls to mind is Captain Beefheart. He had a telepathic relationship with the Magic Band, whoever the players.

Simple Minds' 'Film Theme' plays on a loop as the VIP customers gather in the front four rows. The group shuffle on inauspiciously and Herr Kerr turns on the toned-down version of his stage persona, the epitome of charm. They answer questions about the German influence on their early records and the singer talks articulately and knowledgeably about Hansa Studios and Kraftwerk and krautrock. I think back to myself as a fifteen-year-old kid gazing up at Jim and Charlie at the Glasgow City Hall, squashed at the front, thrilled to be so close. Whatever barrier you perceived between Glasgow and the wider world, Simple Minds made it disappear. If you'd told me then that, forty-four years later, Del Amitri would be opening for Simple Minds in arenas around Europe, I'd have jumped for joy. All those years spent doing what you love. What ridiculous luck. The wall didn't fall. There never was a wall at all.

DAY 82, Frankfurt, Germany

If it's Friday, it must be fucking Frankfurt. First things first, the shorts fit. The April sun is beating on the tarmac around the bus, and I have my Trendy Army Shop shorts on and they're staying up without a belt. Secondly, I establish that I am half an hour's walk from a film museum, so I have a purpose in life. Get a good coffee on the way and I'll be a contented man. I had a bout of nausea in the middle of the night. It was probably as a result of re-watching *Shoah (Second Era)* while travelling over bumpy roads. I had not fully remembered one of the survivors' descriptions of unloading the Auschwitz gas chambers. It is a horrific encapsulation of the moral debauchery of the Third Reich. It is simply disgusting.

The route disappointingly hugs an eight-lane highway, towers of glass and steel gathering in gangs of three or four on either side. There are hills to the north. It could be Salt Lake City. I walk round the chaotic half-circus at the train station, a jungle of trams, roadworks and construction hoardings and on to a pretty pedestrian bridge over the Main, the promenades on both banks flushed in the early spring greening. My first stop is the Städel whose Google Maps blurb has it 'housing a prominent European art collection from the Middle Ages to the present'. The 'prominent' worries me; I take it to mean 'big'. I'm expecting big vulgar things created by artists I've vaguely heard of. I'm not wrong.

But there are some brilliant things among the big showy canvases. There's a beautiful Renoir, *After the Luncheon*: three figures crowded into the frame in an intimate moment, the male looking a bit puggled, trying to light a fag. It's echoed by another painting of three figures, Edvard Munch's *Jealousy*, an explosion of mad colour, the faces lit garishly from below. I love *Portrait of Prince Frederick Charles of Hesse* by Hans Thoma from 1892, looking very 1920s in a red shirt and undetailed green background. There's another, earlier Munch called *In the Tavern*, which appears to depict Thom Yorke in a posh bar dressed as Fagin. There are some below-par Paul Klees, a horrid Picasso portrait in the little Cubist room and two large Chagalls that leave me cold. Best of all is *The Artist's Family* by Otto Dix, portraying the models (especially himself) as a collection of hideous freaks.

I escape in an elevator that I find secreted behind a pillar in a corner and spend some time in what is effectively a private bathroom in the basement. Luxury. You've got to credit German art galleries – they do very nice toilets. That's the thing about the country, the basic stuff works: doors, locks, hinges, latches. They fit components that are built to last. Find me one toilet in the UK without a malfunctioning door lock, busted cistern or fucked sink.

I eventually surface from my sanitary cellar and walk three doors down, along the river, to the German Film Museum. I'm expecting a stylish, noir-black display of early UFA productions and expressionist lighting. It's very dark but not very moody. Much of it is for kids – touchscreen exhibits allowing visitors to re-edit famous footage or fiddle with the soundtrack – nothing you couldn't do in ten minutes with an iPhone. There are the usual displays of crude prototype moving-image technology. Best is a small screening booth showing early films. The Lumière brothers' footage of a train arriving at a station platform and of workers leaving their factory is like stumbling into a carnival of captured ghosts.

On the way out, I get a little stuck behind a group of kindergarten kids. Their minders are having trouble stopping a boy and girl going at one another with flying fists. She's dressed as a Disney princess and he's in a stormtrooper outfit. Exported American violence in action. I stroll back along the Main in the clement afternoon air. Cutting through town, I find myself on Karlstrasse, weaving between the Fentanyl ghouls so reminiscent of our disturbing experience in Vancouver three years ago. It's a boulevard of lost souls in a city of corporate sheen.

The Festhalle is a wonderful old exhibition hall, more than a hundred years old, and is the first of these arenas to have any character. The rest have been faceless black boxes, the only variables being dimensions and capacity. It has a domed ceiling and elegantly curved contours. Of course, it has a Nazi history as well. Hundreds of the city's Jews were driven here during the November pogroms of 1938 and mass transports ran from the hall to concentration camps.

I go looking for off-site food just as the Minds are taking to the stage. I hit the night air to a huge roar from the crowd behind me. What a sound. There's a thin grin of moon high overhead. I walk around the loading compound, cross a plaza and find a basic little bar with outdoor seating. I ask 'Was ist gut?' and the barmaid says 'Everything', before telling me she only has three items available from the fifteen on her blackboard. I plump for Asian noodles. I don't know what it is, but it ain't Asian. But it's hot and filling and dirt cheap, so I'm not moaning. Two tables along, a busker is sipping coffee, his guitar and amp stowed and ready to roll away. His gig is still harder than mine with or without the Parky. Slinging covers all day, exposed to the elements, sucking in traffic fumes and putting up with drunks.

All that and no dressing room. What have I to complain about? Okay, my hand shakes a little.

I sweep back into the venue along wide vacant corridors, buy a Becks zero from a bar kiosk and watch the latter part of the Minds show from just behind the lighting desk. A few people come up to say hello. One guy says, 'I heard about your disease. I wish you all the best.' How nicely put. The bus is parked under a cluster of glass towers lit from within by people living modern lives in a city that has always prided itself on its modernity. I wonder if the addicts are still milling around down on Karlstrasse or whether the working girls have ushered them away. It's easy at the top. Look at that moon grin.

DAY 83, Munich, Germany

Up early, I am. It's summer. We're parked on a patch of waste ground at the side of the venue. I am beshorted for the first time this tour. There's a shopping centre full of cars for some reason. I have a coffee and a tiny croissant filled with a substance so sweet my cheeks clutch together inside my mouth. Today I will mainly be walking in the Englischer Garten. It's a good few hours' walk into the city. Off I go.

I traipse round some playing fields, well-attired ten-year-olds playing six-a-sides to a reasonable standard, through clean suburban cul-de-sacs and into the park. I'm fairly ill today. The shake is bad, the atrial fibrillation is shit, my energy is low. I probably need more sleep. The one o'clock sun sits high in this southern latitude and sears my scalp. I take a seat on a green bench dedicated to Margot and Peter 'ein Himmel voller Sterne' which I guess, from my brief exposure to *Commando* comic– all war, all of the time – has something to do with heaven (iTranslate gives me 'A heaven full of stars'). A church bell clangs far off behind me.

I slog on, eventually reaching the mini brauhaus where I can use the toilet. The park is huge and featureless – flat and samey throughout. I head for home dejectedly. At a local athletic club around the corner from the Zenith, I spot outdoor seating and order some currywurst under sycamore trees in early leaf. Some Bayern Munich fans are milling around, but soon scarper for the 3.30 kick-off against Cologne. My food is violently sweet – a sausage with strawberry jam dusted with curry powder. It's cheap and it's gut. From here, I can hear the rumbling frequencies of Cherisse's drum kit. For some reason, I'm reminded of the scene in *Cabaret* when an innocent fete turns into a fascist knees-up. I must be more original in my associations. The British are obsessed with the Nazis. It's the only thing in history about which we get to feel morally superior. It distracts from our own genocides, our sordid empire of pain.

The crowd are terrific at the Zenith, packed from the get-go in a big, long room with bars along the sides, all standing. Everyone in the group says it's the best yet. I don't tell them that all I could hear for the whole show was 'You're too old, too sick. You're slurring your words, you look stiff, your bass playing is dreadful. When are you going to stop?' I pride myself on simply finishing the shows. So much of what I'm doing doesn't pass muster. I couldn't bear to watch myself. It's best to keep your eyes shut. Pretend it's alright. It's alright.

DAY 84, day off, Dijon, France

I'm roused at seven by something Eric Hobsbawm is saying about Napoleon. It's my tenth run through *The Age of Empire* and I've not been awake for much more than five minutes of it. The sun is coming up. Everything looks like a Cézanne painting. We're outside Besançon in rolling hill country, forested mainly, a few fields. We stop at a service area to wait for our rooms to be ready before setting off around eleven for the thirty-minute drive into Dijon. A warm bright sun illuminates the verdant meadows and pink blossom on the embankments.

My room is satisfyingly garret-like and I open my two dormer windows onto the Jardin Darcy, a handsome little park four floors below. Halfway to today's museum, I'm ensnared by a brasserie so typically French I'm suspicious it might be a film set. The menu is all escargots and boeuf bourguignon. I opt for a Niçoise and frites. The young waiter is winningly proficient and everything I order is on my table in four minutes. He shields my big Perrier within a laminated drinks menu to prevent it warming in the sun.

I soak in the Sunday scene. Toddlers and their grandparents chat like old friends. Surprisingly few folk are drinking wine. There's a stone fountain topped by a bronze female nude and a mini merry-go-round beside it. A slightly frail man resembling a rock star takes the table adjacent to me, giving me a knowing nod. I think we recognise one another as gentlemen who have taken drugs. As Mitch Hedberg has it, 'I used to do drugs. I still do. But I used to, too.' He places his walking stick across his wee table and gets out his pouch of baccy. Two incredibly smart sexagenarian women stand up to leave, dressed in thousands of euros' worth of gear. My neighbour asks if it's okay to smoke and I stupidly interpret him as offering me a puff on a joint. I quickly reverse my negative response when I realise my error. *Mon dieu, comme c'est embarrassant!*

I set off towards a museum through medieval streets roofed in the local toits bourguignons – multicoloured tiles laid in pretty geometric patterns. I pass a man with two identical weird black dogs who look like they're constantly being electrocuted. Maybe they are. I'm waylaid initially by the Musée des Beaux-Arts, housed in the Duke of Burgundy's palace. I don't know if they still have a duke (I'm imagining the guillotine might have had a say in this), but it's a splendid gaff, all lead-lit windows and cobbled courtyards. The first room hosts a bunch of Christian relics of so little interest I flick them the Vs and fuck off.

Up the stairs, I dimly register some rubble from ancient Egypt and a bunch of Renaissance portraits with the slightly lurid countenance of the recently restored. Give me a murky shit-brown canvas covered in cracks. What are these comic-book creations? For some reason I'm forced into a lift, ascending a single floor to materialise in the twentieth century, a smidge of Cubism, some nice 1950s abstracts. Up a flight of steps is a room crowded with ghastly sculptures which might only draw (negative) interest if you installed them among the hydrangeas in a B&Q garden centre. So far these arts ain't very beaux. The top level, in what I see now is a very expensively built modern gallery space within the palace walls, features more woeful statuary and some amusing colourful abstracted still lifes that at least contain a measure of joy. On the stairs as I leave, I'm struck by Jean Messagier's abstract portrait of Louis XIV, which looks exactly like the dirty protest in Steve McQueen's *Hunger*.

Outside in the square, a crowd of OAPs are blocking the entire street because their attention has been caught by a woman dressed as a clown. That's how Nazism begins! That's how easy it is! I escape into the Rude Museum, a collection of enormously boisterous sculptures by François Rude housed in a dilapidated eleventh-century church. I love these things, so bulky and full of bluster. There's Napoleon in black marble sheltering from a storm under a sheet of canvas, a gaunt dead Jesus in his grave clothes, and, most spectacular of all, *Le Départ des Volontaires de 1792*, a gigantic high-relief of writhing bodies topped by a screaming woman with a pterodactyl in her hair and fronted by a naked warrior whose scrotum is bigger than my head. This is proper entertainment.

I pop into the Église Saint-Michel next door, taking a pew as I reminisce. On entering a Catholic church, My Love would always dip two fingers into the nearest font and bless herself. I loved to see that, her connection to this grand mysterious entity being something I'd never had. She said she was hedging her bets. I'm alone with that thought, in this musty building with its high vaulted roof, and am gambling on zero. I know our situation will never improve. I know miracles are the hope of the insane.

I slope back up to the hotel for a sneaky après-midi slumber. At the top of the high street, there's an old cinema of the sort you no longer see in Britain, built into a city block, nested in the fabric of the town centre. Posters advertise five films, all French. When was the last time the equivalent was witnessed in the UK? Was it ever? The French have looked after their film industry; ours is a charity case, so the talent fucks off to the States. The French get Claire Denis and Isabelle Huppert. We get Guy Ritchie and Mr Bean. Hard to tell who the biggest wanker is. Okay, it's Guy Ritchie.

I flop across the double bed, a bright rhombus of sun warming my legs, a cooling breeze curling in over the rooftops. I listen to Erin Rae and drift for an hour. Sleep is the only place I'm safe. I go out for dinner around sunset, eating alone surrounded by the young. I go back to the garret and consider throwing myself out of the window. I decide I'll write 'Fuck it' with a Sharpie on my pillow. I wrestle with whether to add a 'Sorry'. But sorry is so weak. I wouldn't be sorry. I'd be glad to get out of all this suffering on such a pleasant evening.

DAY 85, Dijon, France

I'm sorry to leave the Grand Hôtel La Cloche with its fake art deco fittings and multifarious lighting choices. The carpet too was to my liking, shaggy like a labradoodle and very soothing underfoot. I have an attack of the wobbles as I'm rolling my case to the door, a sure sign things are not right with my psyche. I need a coffee, having had none yesterday. Charlie from the Minds is chatting to Iain beside our parked bus, asking how long we've known each other. I make my excuses ('See you at the enormodome') and leave the two of them on the pavement. Iain is cycling to the venue. He could offer Charlie a backie. The bus takes us through dense suburb to an IKEA zone. A lot of these gigs have been near IKEAs. The Zenith appears, grey and angular, rising from a forest of pylons like a sci-fi fortress. I'd imagine this would be where the baddies live. Inside, everything is painted red. The walls are red, the seats are red, the roof is red. I miss the Cloche already.

There's a little park next door called the Parc de la Toison d'or (the Golden Fleece). I know nothing about this reference, except Jason was a *Blue Peter* cat. Wikipedia helps a little. Jason had help from Medea in stealing the fleece. My mother took me to see a production of *Medea* in Glasgow's Kibble Palace, a Victorian greenhouse in the Botanic Gardens, the park not one block from where I was born. The staging had two long rows of seating on either side of a corridor on which the players strutted. The actor in the title role mesmerised us, walking right up to my mother and imploring her, pleading with her to understand her reasoning for what she was about to do. Those two actors locked eyes, my mother's filled with tears, looking up, in wonder and admiration. And so, we were both convinced that the only logical action was for Medea to slaughter her two children. You don't get shit like that at a pop concert.

I sit on some steps in the sun. There is a carnival of daisies and daffodils in the long grass, clover and lilac too. A lizard scuttles by. Andy and Jim approach, equally bored. Jim heads for the shopping centre, Andy opts for a bench somewhere. He'll have a book. He always has a book. This tour he's been telling me about *Lenin on the Train*, the story of the Bolshevik leader's return from exile to claim power in post-revolutionary Russia. He has also been reading the history of the horse.

It's a Monday-night kind of a crowd and we don't feel we get anything back from them. There's hardly a sound when we take the stage. But the place is full when we finish and there's a hint of a cheer. The whole show was just a battle with Gavin for me. The reminder, the ruiner, the winder-upper, the fucker.

I watch a bit of the Minds; they're sparkling as always. 'This Fear of Gods' gets my hips moving every night. I go to find a zero beer from the foyer, but all the bars are shut, like it's the fucking opera or something. I stay out front 'til 'Promised You a Miracle'; I watch a bit more from stage left. Sarah has some mic issue and I don't want to be in the way, so I dematerialise through the black curtain into the drab normal world, with normal light and normal stuff and normal people doing normal things. The place I'm half alive.

DAY 86, Nantes, France

We're very much not in Nantes. It's forty minutes on a train to any-thing cultural. I can't decide what to do. There doesn't seem to be anything around the venue. There's an IKEA, naturally. I potter and watch time pour away. I eat some toast, drink a coffee, do a cretin's crossword. I slouch back to the bus. I take a pill, the pill takes effect and I make a decision. It's going to be too time-consuming walking twenty minutes to a railway station and sitting on a train for forty minutes. That's over two hours there and back, leaving less than two hours to walk around the city. The ratio of transport to leisure is poor. I'm staying local. I'm going to the fucking shopping centre.

The shopping centre is called Atlantis and is the usual soul-flattening zone – marble tiled floors and undefinable music resounding in the rafters. If it weren't for the copious amount of daylight flooding down from the skylights, I could be back in Uncasville, CT. These complexes are of limited interest to me. I don't wear trainers and I'm not in the market for pastel-coloured clothing or heavily branded scents. Some people dress up to come to these places. I'm tempted to get my left hand done at a nail bar but worry about the language barrier. *No, gloss, non! Verte, oui, mais matte!* Europe has a language problem, sings Herr Kerr in 'I Travel'. Speaking of whom, we hear Jim has a sore throat and has cancelled the Minds' sound-check. I thought all we singers sounded croaky last night. The air in Dijon wasn't great (according to my app) and I bet we all had our hotel windows open. It's a pathetic theory. Sore throats just happen, like earthquakes or twisted ankles.

I realise that if I had all the money in the world, there'd not be a single thing I'd want to buy in this monstrous depot of despair. I sit on a white bench under the atrium. The music speeds up. I think I recognise the voice. It's Coldplay. Fair play, Coldplay. When you've made it to the mall, you've done it all.

I return to the silent sanctuary of my bunk. I read a little more of Patrick deWitt's *The Librarianist*, which I'm savouring. I fall asleep. I'm called for an early soundcheck, so there is even more time to kill before showtime. Andy, Kris and I sit in the slowly darkening dressing room like codgers in a care home. The problem with Mr Kerr's voice has got everyone edgy. The whole circus swirls around his role as ringmaster. I feel guilty that I can sing. When I lost my voice near the start of a three-month tour of the US in 1995, I found myself crying in the foetal position in the shower at the hotel. I was desperately trying to coax my voice back with the humidity. I even took a little humidifier on stage and placed it at the foot of my mic stand. It was no use – nothing was coming out but a ragged whisper and the odd yodel. Al Marks, our field operator for A&M, phoned the LA office the next morning and cancelled all the radio promo we'd been booked to do for the following two weeks. We used to do so much promo on tour. It took twice as much of our time as the soundchecks and shows themselves. Sometimes three radio acoustic performances before soundcheck and two more afterwards. It was mad for a while.

When you're young and you're chasing success, actively having a hit record break, the workload gets absurd. In 1990, I remember finishing club shows in the US at midnight and doing two hours of phone interviews to Australia from my hotel room afterwards. We must have dragged our guitars and accordion to hundreds of shitty radio stations in America in the '90s. I was lucky my voice only gave out that once – though after that episode, I stopped drinking and smoking for the first half of every tour and eventually for whole tours. The last time I had beers every night on a tour was the second two weeks of my 2014 solo US tour with Derek and Showbiz Niz, my erudite accompanist. And that was only possible because US beer was still brewed to a very low alcohol content then. It's all fucked now.

The Nantes folk are kind and pay us a bit of polite attention. I watch a little of the Minds, enough to satisfy myself that Mr Kerr is going to make it through the show. I can see he's digging deep, but he's producing the notes and putting on as a good a show as always. He's more than front, this frontman. I'm relieved for him and the rest of us who sing. I walk out into the cold evening. There's a streak of yellowing sky at the horizon and I turn and look into the ground-floor windows at the back of the arena. The promoter is eating something and staring into a computer. The two catering women, Sarah and Sarah, are sitting together planning tomorrow's menu. It's the first time I've seen either of them off their feet. I watch one of the Sarahs wipe the little blackboard. Another date down, another dawn to come.

DAY 87, day off, Paris

It's 10 a.m. and Iain's getting on his bike for the three-hour cycle to our Paris hotel. We're parked at a service stop in a parc naturel and it's sunny and cool. I take the opportunity to stretch and have coffee and a pain au chocolat in the bright and airy café. I have informed Andy and Jim not to leave without me, but it doesn't stop me keeping a bead on our bus. I've been burnt before. All the trees in the thickly wooded verges are in leaf. Spring happens so quickly. I wonder how green Glasgow will be by Sunday. Suddenly we're in Paris, crossing a pretty bend in the Seine at the Pont de Sèvres. One of the most pleasing things about Paris is that everywhere you go looks like Paris. You lift your head and you can only be here. We turn into Boulevard de Courcelles and the Sacré-Coeur appears on its summit, gleaming like a cloud caught at sunrise. The streets are lined with those spindly trees, watched over by the shallow balconies, with their filigree ironwork and curlicue buttresses. It's obscene to be driving into the centre of the city in our building of a bus, but I can't see how alternative arrangements would produce less carbon. At least there's twelve of us and luggage in a single vehicle.

This being Pigalle, we drive down a row of sex shops and erotic supermarkets. We stop outside Sexodrome Love Store, where I doubt much love is in store. As we're in the land of the double entendre, we unload right there. Jim and I wheel up the street and round the corner to our boutique abode. Très funky. What the tiny rooms lack in space, they make up for in annoying and useless accoutrements that shout: *We're hip!* I find myself spending ten minutes trying to reattach the drive belt to the turntable before I realise how ludicrous it is. The deck gets shunted aside to be replaced by Bluetooth philistinism. My corner window allows dappled light onto the bedspread, shadows of ivy projected onto the muslin curtain moving imperceptibly in the breeze.

I peruse the map doubtfully and, after much thought, decide to just walk vaguely south. What's the worst that can happen? I get myself in the mood with a bit of Bob Dylan's first (comedy) album, the one where he's puffing at his mouth organ like a drowning donkey. It's very cheering. I bump into Iain in the foyer who says getting through the Périphérique on his bike was crazy. I tell him I'm just going to wander haphazardly and he says, 'best place for it'. I turn a corner and find a microphone shop. I have never heard of a microphone shop. I daren't enter, even if a microphone will be the last bit of kit I'll have any use for. Next door is a jigsaw shop.

This might be the red-light area, but it's well pukka. I try to follow a sewing motion, down and to the left, down and to the right. I pass a dental school embedded in a cliff face of apartments and come to a street of upmarket boucheries, charcutiers, traiteurs, fromageries and chocolatiers. There are minute vintage clothes shops that look impossibly expensive. A left takes me down a street of private art galleries, antique shops and two-chair hairdressers. It starts to rain and I don the gear: waterproof shell, hat given to me in Inverness two years ago by a lovely woman with a knitwear shop. I nose into a few cafés seeking shelter and something French, finding, at third try, the perfect spot, a corner brasserie with the *prix fixe* blackboard menu. I order an entrée and a plat, not entirely certain what each dish contains. I speak broken French to the quite beautiful waitress and she replies in perfect, American-accented English. I apologise for my lameness, but keep trying and am thanked for it.

The entrée is, as I suspected, mushrooms with something green, in this case string beans. It also features ham, sneaky strips of it hiding among the vegetables. My plat is not, as I thought, pork but fish. It's perfectly cooked and comes with a vibrant tomato sauce and rice run through with lightly sautéed scallions. It's all so simple and easy. Zero pretension. Locals come and go, taking coffees at the bar and indulging in casual gossip with the barman. A businessman with two phones exudes a quiet loathing. An English couple arrive, eat and depart in the time I am savouring the essentially Parisian nature of it all: the floor tiles, the cobbles, the five-storey buildings with those high dormer windows set into the steep roofs so the city has a thousand eyes.

I walk in the rain for a bit and duck into the Museum of Romantic Life to get dry. It's free! The French are good at free. I have my bag checked in a see-through tent set across an alleyway leading to a sumptuous little courtyard beautifully planted and dominated by a gorgeous two-storey house, painted cream with green shutters. It's a hidden Shangri-La of climbing plants and flowering shrubbery. I ascend the weather-worn steps up to the house. The attendants are forbiddingly reverent. Everyone within is whispering and creeping about as if a great figure from history were sleeping upstairs and I fight the urge to fart. I have no idea what this place is about and I am not inspired to find out. Someone arty lived here, I'm guessing, and there are a great many references to George Sand. There are some dull portraits and morbid sculptures of a woman's disembodied hands in a horizontal display case (it turns out the arm is Sands', the hand is Chopin's). I take a bench outside as two friends from the US greet one another as if for the first time in years. 'So, we both got the denim memo,' says the man. 'Hey gang, me too!' I should have interjected. I spot a WC sign as I leave. I'm not ashamed to say that, in the Musée de la Vie Romantique, I had a shit.

I keep walking downhill until it flattens out and gets a bit London-like. Every now and then, you turn a corner onto a narrow street to be met with some massive and important building blocking the end of the road. I trek back up the hill to the hotel, sitting outside with a coffee opposite the Dirty Dick, a Polynesian-themed cocktail bar. Gav the guitar tech comes by and Gavin waves him hello. Up in my room, the metro rumbles from deep below in the city's bowels like a giant stirring from a century-long sleep.

DAY 88, Paris, France

My great friend Pol Wilson arrived last night and we had escargots and steak frites at a bistro two doors from my hotel. Gavin was dancing uncontrollably at the excitement of it all. My brain found it hard to keep up, unused to socialising (for four months) with Gavin and Pol vibrating at a higher frequency than I could manage. Pol gave me a job in 1986 when I returned from our insane make-or-break US tour, broke and in danger of getting evicted. He turned me from an ex-chef into a very decent waiter, got me back on my feet and was a magnificent boss. He introduced me to My Love and, with his wife Rosie, has been my longest and most loyal friend. We don't get enough time together, so last night was beautiful. Even with zero-alcohol beer.

Sometimes I think I just dumped her like a bag of rubbish at the care system's door. Sometimes I think if you love someone that much, you'd never let it happen. This one's broken – bring me another. The heel that I am. The heel that can't live without her, but insists on doing so. I think, *Justin – this was all of your design. You failed to look after her, accidentally broke her and now are looking for a way out.* That vermin that is love, which creeps under the doors of your ribcage and liquidises your heart. What does love matter, what does it mean? What is your duty and what is your scheme? I despise myself for letting this happen to her. Under my watch. Sometimes we hold hands, we two failures, and everything is alright. I don't care about the guilt. I care about the love. Love that could no longer maintain without the extraordinary support of the system and our community. Without them, I'd be a twenty-four-hour-a-day carer. And both of us would be destroyed. What a dreadful settlement. What a dreadful time.

My Love asks after our cat, asks after me. Not a thought for herself, glued to a wheelchair, bored beyond belief. The hero should save the day. But what does he have left to save when so much has been taken away? Except for love. The love is here to stay.

In the morning, I dump my kit on the bus and jump back off to spend more time in the city. The first thing Maps throws up is a jazz museum. Ideal. I hike uphill to Rue des Abbesses and consume the obligatory coffee and croissant outside a café. I look at the myriad flakes I leave on my little dish. What happens to all these croissant flakes? How many end up fattening the pigeons and the rats? The passers-by wear expensive camel-coloured coats, walk expensive dogs and trail expensive children. Every block has two trendy optician's selling the same mildly eccentric designs. Quirky bourgeois. It's a pretty route, up and down leafy flights of steps to a museum which is very much fermé. Shut up, shutters down, nothing doing.

I set course for the venue, another Zenith, no doubt on another godforsaken hill in a retail hinterland. The long straight route starts to get dull, so I divert south through a Senegalese neighbourhood, stopping in a local park to watch some kids play football and some men play checkers on gridded tables. I'm taken back to the chaotic opening day of the France '98 World Cup. We'd been Eurostar'ed into Paris the day before the Scotland vs Brazil game. We were doing a feature for *Q* magazine and two Radio 1 acoustic performances of

'Don't Come Home Too Soon' (they did). Our now-manager, Andy P, who was running A&M's press department at the time, had to find six tickets for the match at twenty-four hours' notice because the promised allocation from the commercial operation running Scotland's non-sporting affairs never showed up. The tickets were for competition winners, one of whom was the eight-year-old boy pictured on our single sleeve who was in Paris with his granddad expecting to be at the game. This sent the record company into a panic, recruiting London ticket touts to source seats on the black market in Paris. The touts trawled the bars looking for Scotland fans willing to part with their tickets for cash. The asking price was £2,000 per ticket. An accountant was duly dispatched from London with twelve grand in a briefcase, the tickets were sourced and a potential publicity disaster avoided. The only problem was that some of the tickets had the original purchaser's name printed on them for security reasons. Iain and I gave our tickets to the *Q* journalist and photographer. They had to pretend to be Mr and Mrs Roux.

The second Radio 1 performance took place in a scrappy square near the stadium and, after hanging around having a laugh with Catatonia, we got involved in a massive Scotland fans versus local French Algerian kids football free-for-all. Beers, musicians and a kickabout. What a perfect day.

I come down the hill from the peace of the city park into a scrum of humanity on the Boulevard de la Chapelle. It's a shock to suddenly be jostling and weaving. I find a café for sanctuary and look out across the boulevard where a low-lying block of shops reveals the three towers and dome of the Sacré-Coeur. Paris never lets you forget where you are. And I haven't seen the Eiffel Tower once. La Chapelle takes me through a North African neighbourhood with its pastry stands and moped workshops, across two wide rivers of railway tracks and left onto the Quai de la Seine running along the wide canal. I stop by a little marina and watch some men play boules. They take careful measurement of the ball's weight before each throw. When the metal balls strike together, they make a clacking sound, like a robot clicking its fingers. Some of the men throw slow and high with lots of backspin, some throw low and aggressively, trying to force an opponent away from the jack. They have telescopic sticks with magnets to pick up their boules without stooping. I get to the venue and follow the what3words locator. A security guard calls out to me.

'VIP?'

'Non! Artiste! Artiste!'

He waves me on.

DAY 89, Cournon-d'Auvergne, France

I have a long, long sleep. I do not want to go home. I don't want to go back to seeing My Love imprisoned by fate. I don't want to deal with all the hellishness around it. I do my stupid exercises in the back lounge. I look at the map. It's too arduous a journey to go into nearby Clermont-Ferrand. Besides, the Minds have cancelled another VIP party, so we will soundcheck early. I nose around the venue car park. I can't see anywhere to go. There's a little hill on the other side of the motorway and I wonder if I might be able to climb that. I note that Clermont-Ferrand is surrounded by a chain of dormant volcanos. I look up and there is the largest, the Puy de Dôme, tipped with snow.

I head for the nearest hill along newly laid cycle paths, up into the village of Pérignat-les-Sarliève, with its re-paved streets and elegant glass bus shelters. It's all very spiffy. In fifteen minutes, I hit a dirt track, butterflies dabbling along the path in front of me, finding myself elevated enough to peep through a hedge and view the city spread out around the base of all this tectonic activity like spilled stew. I pause by a scrubby slope to watch a small herd of chestnut horses graze. A military jet streaks through the wide flat valley. Another follows minutes later, carving silently through the mountain air followed by a thunderous groan. A lizard skulks into the undergrowth where something heavier, mammalian, rustles unseen.

I come to an impasse. I can move left, right or back down, but my way upwards is blocked by a wall of dense wild forest. I make an attempt to chop through but it's useless. I'm frustrated. The summit is only a few hundred feet vertically and maybe a ten-minute climb away. I sit on a boulder by the side of the track and inhale the sweetness of the country air. A creature behind me, presumably a bird, is making exactly the same noise the boules made yesterday when striking one another. It's unnerving, like a demented shepherd boy approaching while clicking two pebbles together. I hear a rooster hiccup below. If I concentrate, I can hear at least ten specific types of birdsong.

I'm coming down the hill with the sunlight streaming past my shoulders. Ahead on the horizon there's a line of snow frosting a mountain plateau. The image comes to me of My Love doing physiotherapy in her room and suddenly pushing the exercise ball away in tears of despair and I hide my face in my hands, hoping tears come now when I'm alone on this hill and not in some other unforeseen moment.

Herr Kerr is very unwell. A doctor is in attendance, oxygen standing by. Rumours and counter rumours have been circling all day. The backstage area is morgue-like with dread of a cancellation. All these people depending on him, this bandwagon of trucks and buses, the thousands of expectant ticket holders – I know how it weighs on you. And when you're sick? It's grim and there's no way out – you have to get through it or call it. I watch half an hour and Kerr's effort is extraordinary, he somehow pulls it all up from inside himself. I don't imagine anyone in the crowd will suspect anything's wrong.

We bus out early, 10 p.m. I cross my fingers the frontman gets through to the finish. I've been listening to the Dylan studio albums in order since the day off in Paris. Tonight, I play the second side of *Bringing It All Back Home*, all that power, all that talent. As I cue *Highway 61 Revisited*, the bus groans and pulls out, just as that first snare hit sounds. Lights swirl about in the blackness outside and we waddle onto the highway bound for the city of Milan. How does it feel? It feels good not to be going home.

DAY 90, Milan, Italy

I'm in need of land facilities, so I'm dressed and off bus at nine-thirty. The venue is very much the police headquarters in *Blade Runner*. I walk up an exterior ramp to take a view of the mountains to the north and west – Hannibal's Alps! The snow is dazzling and the sky nothing short of azure. I have friends in town and head to MUDEC, an art complex in a converted factory where I am to liaise with Damien and Elspeth. I catch a train at 10.56 (don't mention Benito), departing on time. I sit opposite the trendiest-looking sixty-something man I've ever seen. He has swept-back grey hair and a perfectly clipped beard – not too long, not too neat – and is wearing a lightweight khaki suit, no socks and deck shoes. His skin is dark olive oil and his sunglasses vintage. All he's carrying is a book and a phone.

I emerge from the underworld into a calm, crowded residential neighbourhood and follow the blue dots to the museum. The sun stings the skin on the back of my neck with the comfort of a concerned friend. I wander into a courtyard, pulled by a stream of people who are viewing something sponsored by Toyota. The corporate gobbledegook written in English on a banner is enough to dissuade me and I turn tail. There is a queue for a Swiss design place. Something is happening here and I don't know what it is…

I pass more and more heavily branded temporary exhibition spaces. Finally, I spot a lamppost pennant – Milano Design Week. The venues have the anti-appeal of LA nightclubs – doormen in black Armani, outdoor carpet, velvet ropes. Apart from the word 'design', it is impossible to ascertain the delights within. So I remain without. Besides, these places are crowded and the punters coming out don't look too impressed. I find what I think is MUDEC and walk into what looks like an IKEA, lots of boxy brightly coloured furniture with price tags. It's too busy for my tender disposition and I sit on a yellow thing before scarpering. Back on the street, I ponder my next move, deciding to head back towards the station when I realise my error. I'd missed the actual MUDEC's main entrance by ten metres. The place I'd mistaken it for turns out to have been a pop-up IKEA show.

We enter the Martin Parr exhibition. It's consistently superb. I was not familiar with his early black and white work, the examples of which here are pitch-perfect. One delicious scene features a married couple facing one another over a B&B breakfast table, he puffing on a column of ash, she regarding her nails with bitterness. Elspeth remarks that now they would both be on their phones. The shots from New Brighton are brilliant, his compositions and timing a serious delight. The three of us note that, other than the photographs of the spoilt youth of the Oxbridge set, the pieces are non-judgmental but highly political. He has a voice and it's very impressive. We run short of time so don't get to see the permanent collection (which I'm disappointed about), but lunch with five of My Love's friends is urgently needed oxygen for my soul.

I watch a bit of the Minds four songs in and they're incredible. The energy is thrilling, they are positivity radiant. Herr Kerr throws caution to the wind with no tomorrow to concern him. The venue throbs with their energy, made in Glasgow. Without Orange Juice, without Simple Minds, we simply wouldn't have had the juice. I would never have had the courage. We built our city on their rocks.

I careen into a long drunken night from dressing room to bus to airport hotel bar. I somehow make it to the gate in the morning, but sleep through the boarding. Damn. A hellish day ensues, waiting in various European airports on the tortuous route home. Another drunken calamity. Another day alive in the only world I'll know.

DAY 91, Dubai, UAE

I'm tucking into a salmon ceviche in the Emirates lounge at Glasgow Airport. The room is filled with light, hushed but for the tinkling of cutlery and china at the buffet. If my fellow travellers are doing business, they are very casually dressed. Like the salmon. At short notice, we have foolishly agreed to replace Deacon Blue at some Euros-themed gig in Dubai. Tomorrow night sees the opening match of the championships and the Scotland men's football side are to take on Germany. We will be the light entertainment on stage before the heavy kicking starts on screens. We're pumping obscene amounts of carbon into the air to frolic in an absolute monarchy. I could say I was railroaded into doing this show, but I'm here and I'm guilty of all charges: hypocrisy, greed and moral turpitude. There's a prayer room next to the immaculately tiled toilets (with showers). Perhaps I should ask for forgiveness. What do you call it when you knowingly transgress? It is a crime.

I sit in the darkness of a cubicle; its energy-saving light has clicked off. I wave my hand like a magician and achieve illumination. A stall for ablutions stands by the marble sinks. I am in the first world feeling greasy and unclean. I'm a heathen and a barbarian. I can't even pretend to be on a mission of cultural import. I'm a cheap act committing a heinous one.

We have an irregular backline crew, Brian, Buddy and Gav being otherwise detained by work with bands who have more gigs in their diaries than we. The calm, laconic Hugh has stepped in before, but Davis is new to us. He has large ruddy sideburns shaved to a point. I'm jealous of their lack of grey. Greyness starts slowly, but completes its invasion quickly. When I was drunk and high a few weeks ago, I looked into the bathroom mirror. On returning to the company in my living room, I appeared haunted and upset. My friend Aldo asked me what was wrong. 'Mirror.' I replied. 'Never do that.' he advised.

The plane is some enormous Airbus thing I've never seen before. It looks fat and ridiculous with two rows of windows, upstairs/downstairs. We business cunts are, naturally, up top. 'My' stewardess introduces herself and asks how she should pronounce my surname. I'm momentarily flummoxed. I want to say, 'Oh, don't bother with that. Just call me Your Highness.' She wafts her china doll-like manicured hands in front of me, pointing out my seat's features. There's a huge touchscreen set in walnut veneer. There's a tablet and a remote control. There's a mini-bar. I can't cope. What do I start fiddling with first? Frank Sinatra is singing 'You Make Me Feel So Young' on the cabin sound system. A pair of stainless-steel tongs appears proffering a hot towel. I swaddle my face and smell lemongrass. Families are being ripped apart on the ground in Gaza while I will dine finely in the kingdom of the air. We are attended to by a platoon of petite women in perfectly applied make-up. We are to live like emperors for the duration, it appears. In the menu, 'Words From Our Chef' explains what they like to do with aubergines in Arabia. I ponder what we like to do with Mars Bars in Scotland. Half of the menu is written in Arabic. It looks beautiful – flowing and decorative.

I select the tail-cam and watch the plane's nose tilt up into the sky while feeling the monstrous push from behind. It's the quietest take-off I've ever experienced, surreal and thrilling. As we ascend into the murk of low cloud, the camera ices up, making abstract patterns on my screen. It's like lying under a pane of glass during heavy snowfall. I click my ears and the cabin sounds come alive – cabinet doors clunking open in the galley, passengers clearing their throats, the rustling of packaging. The engines below emit a muted hum. Pastel-coloured lighting fades up in the frets of the ceiling. The travellers are stirring, fussing with their handbags, unfastening and stretching, oblivious to the seatbelt signs forbidding unbuckling. Suddenly my screen flashes violently from black to white. I think the tail-cam is on the fritz. I take to the bog. The toilet seat too is walnut. And there is a window. A window in the bog! And a full-length mirror. It shows a middle-aged man in denim with bad skin and lank, thinning hair. I have forgotten to heed the Advice of Aldo. I sit on my throne in the attitude of prayer, sailing like a speeding bullet through the world.

DAY 92, Dubai, UAE

I slumber long and deeply after finally getting a room key around 3 a.m. I raise myself at 1 p.m. and crack the drapes. Not much to see, just a wall of bland domestic towers such that you might expect to see in a beach resort. I can discern nothing with any style. For a city which has been in a frenzy of construction over the last thirty years, it is amazingly faceless. It's as if someone has randomly selected a bunch of Hyatt and Marriott hotel buildings from minor middle-American cities and dumped them all in the Persian Gulf. It's my second time here and my fleeting impression is the same. What is its character? Where is its heart? I cannot say. I browse the map. I see 'The World' artificial archipelago is still uninhabited. It is a conglomeration of desert islands just off the coast of a megalopolis and a monument to real estate hubris. I smile at this.

I find Kris waiting in the lobby for the limo. After informing me that his daughter Rosie is currently in hospital with suspected meningitis, he divulges that since our last Simple Minds show in Milan, he visited his GP complaining of breathlessness and heartburn. Within minutes, he was blue-lighted to hospital and fitted with two stents, having been told he'd already suffered several minor heart attacks. Heavens to Betsy! Kris says he gets teary when he thinks about the exceptional team of NHS staff who were waiting to whisk him into theatre. One minute he was having mild difficulty walking up the steps in Montmartre, the next they're saving his life with keyhole surgery in Cornwall. Now he's on a cocktail of drugs and feeling better than he has done in years. Kris wanted to tell us face to face so as not to worry us. He does look well. I worry about Rosie. The older we get, the more perilous each tour becomes. By late afternoon, she is out of the woods and heading home.

The soundcheck is a frantic affair. New crew, no rehearsal, problems with the hired gear and an inexperienced monitor engineer. We run over by about ten minutes. Take a deep breath and think of Scotland...

Back at the hotel, I open the curtains onto the ugly edifices of the Dubai skyline. It's still insufferably hot outside. There are a few pedestrians making the short walk from building to vehicle. There are no streets – just ramps and slip roads and service bays. The whole city is a survival suit bolted onto Mars.

We walk onstage in the Coca-Cola Fanzone to a muted reception from the few hundred or so ex-pat types who have dressed for the occasion in football shirts and scraps of tartan. There are some kilts. It doesn't feel like a party, unless it's for the twenty-first birthday of some millionaire's daughter that everybody hates. The gig's one positive aspect is that Gavin is remarkably well behaved and only fucks up my bass playing twice. We come back on for the encore after a minute's silence. I chant 'We want more' from the wings to no avail.

I wake up at 4.58 for a 5 a.m. departure. I'm in the van by seven minutes past the hour. An orange disc of sun hangs at the end of the freeway – there is a fire at the centre of our system. Dubai's weirdly '80s-style architecture drifts past on both sides like bad CGI from a cheap TV version of Orwell's *1984*. It's a penal colony designed by Donald Trump during a bout of food poisoning. It's a colossal folly, a carpet of crap. It's the future and the future is hell.

DAY 93, Scarborough, UK

We have overnighted from Glasgow on a shabby bus that's kitted out in executive grey with blue LED piping. The upstairs back lounge looks like the emergency boardroom on Stalin's train, a place where disappearances are to be decided upon. I slide out of my stuffy bunk at 10 a.m. and peer out between Venetian blinds. The sunshine is raining straight down onto mature trees. I see a stage and a forklift, hard hats and hi-vis tabards. I count the hours on my watch face and decide 11 a.m. is the optimum time to drop my first pill. I slap on a nicotine patch and do my pathetic exercise regime on the woolly shag pile (also grey). Once sufficiently stimulated, I shall seek caffeine and Scarborough itself. What delights await?

We are finishing touring for a while with four shows, again supporting Simple Minds in small English coastal resorts. I'm calling it the Seaside Special. At last – the end of the pier. I meet Steve, our grizzly Scottish driver. He seems like a well-seasoned man and directs me to the 'bollocks', by which I infer he means catering and dressing rooms. The outdoor stage is wedged up against a narrow strip of marshland beyond which lies a narrow-gauge train track. The little train toots as a few elderly day trippers get dragged past sitting inside open-air cars and looking underwhelmed. I prepare for a day of being underwhelmed and look forward to it. I take coffee and a banana in the pleasant marquee backstage and plot a journey to the beach. A local crew lad banters with a caterer in a broad Yorkshire accent. The sky leadens and I pop back to the bus to pack a waterproof and a knitted hat.

As I walk off site, I am suddenly hit by the stench of seaweed as a scrap of muddy sea appears before me. The rusted pillar of a defunct cable car stands sentry on the path. I hear birdsong and the shush of waves. I come to the North Bay, perhaps a mile wide, bounded to the north and south by low grassy cliffs. Vibrantly painted beach huts sit above the sea wall looking out to the horizon. Norway is over there somewhere. There's a scattering of tourists and local dog walkers sauntering along the promenade. At the water's edge, a family of four in silhouette inspect a sandcastle which perfectly echoes the ruin on the hill beyond. At the road, I stop at a sign and spot a sponsor's logo: Scarborough Art Gallery. That'll do. Set controls for the heart of the culture.

I climb a path that takes me up the rise at the back of the bay. Sitting on a wooden memorial bench (Kath Haigh S.R.N. 1950–2013), I survey the scene below. Children and dogs gambol in the shallow surf looking remarkably like figures from an L.S. Lowry painting. The wind wraps thick salty air around me. A group of novice bodyboarders tentatively paddle into the brown waves below, as a single seagull keens overhead as mournful as a grieving mother. The sun burns through the canopy and caresses the back of my neck. The sound of a barking dog floats up against the massive inexorable racket of the sea meeting land.

Off the front, I hike up an ugly road of brick terraces, coming to a row of shops. Hints of the town's past show through in random snatches; on a gable end, the faded white lettering of Trafalgar Boarding House is still legible, while above an old newsagent's door, I spot a sign for Woodbine cigarettes. Everywhere paint is peeling, gutters and shutters rusting. I pass the YMCA Theatre ('Pantomimes, Variety, Plays, Musicals, Ballet, Opera, Comedy') and notice a poster advertising 'Back to the Decades – Celebrating the music of the '80s, '90s, '00s and '10s'. We '60s and '70s music fans are too decrepit to cater to, I guess. An Irish pub sits between a casino and a carpet shop, a beauty parlour squeezed between a tattooist and a second-hand games store.

The buildings become a little more grand as I approach the town centre. I stop in a leafy square overlooking the South Bay. There's a small big wheel and a funicular tramway leading down to the beach. I come to a stunning yellow sandstone, early-Victorian crescent looking onto a beautiful garden, beyond which lies the lovely art gallery. I'm greeted warmly by the receptionist and talked through the exhibits. First is a show by Scarborough photographer Derrick Santini, whose distinctly average portraits of local young adults in the first room begin the expected underwhelming. But the celebrity portraits are better – a decent black and white shot of Jarvis Cocker smoking a fag and a very good frame of One Direction running along a street looking like children. There's a terrible Judi Dench beside a brilliant colour shot of Sleaford Mods hanging upside down in an abattoir. I pass Pam Hogg giving the camera the vicky. I wonder how she is.

There's a roomful of Alan Ayckbourn memorabilia, recalling one of the London trips my mother took me on to go to the theatre.

I remember enjoying Ayckbourn's *Bedroom Farce* at the age of fourteen. My mother – a professional actress before having her children – was keen for me to act. I had lead parts in a couple of school productions: the lawyer in *The Winslow Boy*, and I played one of the two critics in Tom Stoppard's *The Real Inspector Hound*. On the second night of the latter, I made a major error, answering the first phone call in Act One with the dialogue for the second call in Act Two, thus cueing the last section of the play. The rest of the cast gamely carried on and the play abruptly finished prematurely. Thinking on his feet, the sound guy cued the ringing phone again, whereupon we performed the middle of the play last and walked off. The whole thing was so confusing anyway that no one noticed and my drama teacher was very forgiving. But I still sweat about it.

Upstairs, I find some pot ugly nineteenth-century landscapes and a ridiculous diorama of stuffed seabirds beside a wooden peep show from the 1930s. Another room of post-war painting is equally uninspiring. But the building is wonderful, each room laid out around a central balcony connecting the two levels elegantly. I find a pleasant café in a pretty annex next door, gazing onto verdant parkland through floor-to-ceiling windows. The thin spire of St Martin-on-the-Hill pokes above the tree line. I hack at a tough cinnamon swirl with a blunt wooden knife. I have seen more culture in an afternoon here than I could find in a week in Dubai. Some undefinable thought crosses behind the screen in my mind that separates my consciousness from the darkness beyond and Gavin shakes with a sudden violence. The first sign today. I count the hours to my next pill and count the days to my next drink, next cigarette, the next time I can spend not giving a fuck about it all – the disease, My Love in hell, the dead and the dying and the slow descent. Today the tremor, tomorrow the quake. Today is simply heaven.

DAY 94, Llangollen, UK

I wake at midday in rural north Wales. The sun is out, I put my boots on. The venue is a cute country arts centre and the many security staff at every corner of every staircase and corridor are so friendly I suspect they're evangelical Christians. It's a little too much before coffee which, I am horrified to discover, consists of a bucket of Nescafé and an urn. How dispiriting. I pass through a ticket office hut to gain the main drag and promptly drift into the overgrown graveyard around St John's Church. I pass by an Eleanor Dove and stop at an ornamental stone commemorating Llewelyn Lloyd Jones, the equivalent, surely in these parts, of Jock McTavish. Poor little Llewelyn, dead aged seven years and nine months in 1864, one hundred years before my birth. Llewelyn Lloyd Jones of Llangollen, murdered by a surfeit of L's. The grass around the graves is shoulder height. Someone needs to get active with a scythe.

I sit on a bench and the sun beats through my denim jacket with surprising strength. A pigeon hoots despondently as Simple Minds' bass drum thumps in the near distance. I need to fortify myself with a walk and caffeine before facing the God Squad again. Let's be off. As I pass back through a colonnade of tombstones, I reflect on the lack of any markers left to memorialise my parents – my sisters and I having no sentimental attachment to such trifles. Their daily appearances in our minds is testament enough.

I wander into a junk shop opposite, housed in a red-brick deconsecrated chapel. A Liverpudlian man in his seventies recognises me, having been introduced by our former tour manager, Quinner, in 2014. He mentions being with his wife back then and is struck dumb for a few moments, giving the clear impression she walks among us no more. I leave him to his reverie without further enquiry. I find a basket of 'women's sunglasses', buying four at two pounds a pair. I have learned far too late in life that all sunglasses are disposable. Once understood, one should never spend more than a fiver. Like cigarettes – as soon as they're placed on a pub table, they're not coming home.

The town is tourist-quaint, set around a river running through low green hills. The place is crawling with pensioners in shorts and T's, many sporting those alpine sticks that denote the ageing rambler. The high street is all picturesque pubs, cute tea rooms and camping shops. I'm guessing these docile visitors are from nearby English settlements, swarming into Wales to get a taste of the Celtic. There's a preponderance of old men on new bicycles, wrinkled retirees desperately staving off a coronary. I sip a half-drinkable Americano outside what claims to be a bistro but is fooling no one. The first item on the menu, below the full English, is scampi and chips. A man stops to say hello. We met in Sydney Airport a year ago. He had been visiting his sister. I briefly consider Sydney Sister as a song title. I've invoked the city in song before and won't better it, I reckon.

A staircase within the café leads to an enormous second-hand bookshop and I drift to the film aisle. There are at least twenty different volumes on Greta Garbo, three on the wonderful Sarah Miles. I buy a hardback Katharine Hepburn biography, reasoning that it will lead me to hitherto undiscovered performances. Since My Love was stricken, I have eschewed our former diet of trash TV and politics. *Question Time* and *I'm a Celebrity* are no fun at all without the funniest woman in the world hurling profane bon mots. I've tried to emulate her withering commentaries, but the house feels emptier as a result. So instead, I watch Hollywood movies of the '30s and '40s, and bask in the wit and grace of the writing, acting and direction. I'm currently falling asleep to an audiobook life of Howard Hawks. The meathead who narrates is so useless it's hilarious. Misreadings, mispronunciations, fluffed names all left unedited. If I could figure out the procedure, I'd ask for my money back. But the book has taken me to parts of Hawks's oeuvre I'd not previously seen. His are heart-warming films, full of declared love between men and romantic battles of wit between men and women. His Westerns hardly ever step out of the saloon or the parlour, and his attention to actors in supporting roles is formidable. He's the auteur of the soundstage.

I follow a leafy path along the river, meeting a Welshman and his teenage son up from Carmarthenshire for tonight's show. Their accents are soft and mellifluous, like the waters of the River Dee itself. Men come by in work gear and begin scrubbing bird shit from the ornate iron lampposts. Once again, bathos. Hikers and their sticks click by, mounting up their tallied steps. Ahead lies a thickly wooded hill over-looking a pleasing bend in the river. This is a very managed kind of wildness, somewhere between the manicured neatness of rural England and a Highland village.

Back on the A-road that leads to the gig, a man leaps out of a black Range Rover waving with enthusiasm. He's Alan, another Scouser, and, after asking about my health, announces he has four months to live. Throat cancer has metastasised. He looks tanned and fit. He tells me that, since his terminal diagnosis, he's ditched all the meds and is taking cat worming tablets. By all appearances, this seems to be working. His wife takes our photograph, the afflicted in one another's arms, and we part with a cheerful 'See you on the other side!'. God bless bravado, it helps until it doesn't. This is the fascinating thing about being publicly ill. People open up. Last night, while watching the Minds, a young mother told me about her son's tremor and her certainty that he has MS. I think she just wanted to share. It's not like the Ghastly Affliction makes me an expert, but I guess you can bet on my having a level of empathy I might have previously lacked.

I take my former seat in the graveyard, sunbathing in a field of the dead. Beyond the roof of a pretty, pink-brick Victorian villa, the ruin of Castell Dinas Brân sits atop a mount. There are no ghosts, only remnants in stone.

DAY 95, Margate, UK

I appear to be in Dismaland. There is fake turf, bits of broken rides, a rusting shipping container. Alas, we are backstage at Dreamland, a fun park hanging off the back of Margate. Perhaps this was Banksy's inspiration. Iain guides me to the services, our pleasant dressing room located in a wooden hut that looks on to an unpainted wooden roller-coaster. I sense here, too, inspiration for Emin's version, the one that crashes into a wall. Our Tracey, the Margate enfant terrible, the great YBA survivor.

We were recording *Can You Do Me Good* around uber-hip Old Street circa 1999. The tech bubble was yet to burst and east London was awash with wankers of every description. City boys in Savile Row duds, young mums on bone-rattler bikes with baguettes sticking out of their front baskets, artistic types with no socks. It was very grimy and very hip. There was an exhibition at the White Cube gallery collecting a few works by the stars of the scene, the brilliant Chapman brothers' *Disasters of War* among them. But the piece de resistance was Emin's *Everyone I Have Ever Slept With 1963–1995*. I entered that little tent and sat among the tenderly appliquéd names – Mother, Billy Childish, Tracy Horn. I'd seen her notorious *My Bed* at the Turner Prize exhibition previously and quickly discounted it. Steve McQueen's amazing video pieces (including the awesome *Deadpan*) won that year. But the tent was something else. I sat for a few minutes within, intensely moved. I can count on one hand artworks that have had such a profound emotional effect on me. I found myself in tears. On the wall opposite hung one of Emin's neon slogans. I can't remember the text, but it left me cold. But the tent alone cements her status as one of the giants of that feverish era. It has the same emotional punch as Gaudí's enormous Jesus of Nazareth lettering at the rear of the Sagrada Familia. Both pieces are acts of adoration and speak elo-quently of love. The Emin tent went up in smoke in the 2004 Momart warehouse fire and she has refused to remake it. Take everyone's word for it. It was astonishing.

Emin's fame has put Margate on the map. I wander out to find it. The seafront is reassuringly shithole-adjacent. Crumbling, peeling facades, deserted amusement arcades, a single, tatty tower block. I sit on a seagull-shit-encrusted bench in an overgrown triangle of park surrounded by grunting traffic and look on to a turquoise sea, banded dark green with kelp beds. It's gloriously grim. A codger with a hack-ing cough splutters behind me. I make for the Turner, passing some old mod blokes with faces of tanned leather. Glory was it to ruck with the bikers in the '60s.

The gallery sits on a rise on the front. I can't describe the building because it is merely a white void against the sky. A square, pointy void. I find nothing of interest on the ground floor. White walls hung with indifferent art, poured concrete floors. Upstairs is a roomful of angry abstracts from the early '60s by Chicagoan Ed Clark. There's a pretty self-portrait done before Ed 'embraced abstraction', according to the blurb. At first, I see nothing but violent frustration, but as I sit in the gallery's centre, the five large canvasses grow on me. They're of their time, but there is a singular voice in them, and it's not irrelevant. That voice suits my bleak mood today. I'm harassed because I have friends to hook up with, both of whom have arranged to take my photograph. This means I need to find somewhere to shave in the funfair. Shaving, if Gavin is not calm, is often less ablution than act of humiliation. Sometimes it's a scene of self-mutilation.

A second room displays Clark's later work from the late '70s – softer and calmer, using an elliptical shape as a framing motif. The colours have become muted and you sense seascapes and sunsets going on in the horizontal lines. I don't 'like' these paintings, but I admire their originality. In Room 4, works from the '80s through to the zeroes show another tonal shift. I love an untitled abstracted landscape from 2005 which is very reminiscent of Howard Hodgkin's bravura swashes of strong colour. Hodgkin's son, Sam, directed the video for 'Stone Cold Sober' for us in 1989. Another fine soul whose path we never crossed again. I really like Room 4.

I take coffee and quiche in the café, looking out on visitors sunning themselves on the ironic striped deckchairs scattered about the concourse. Texts come in. Both photographer friends have arrived at the same time. I put Colin – this volume's cover photographer – back to after soundcheck and move Geoff up to 3 p.m. Geoff has me stand, lean and sit on a concrete block in a car park outside the Dreamland fence. I pull my usual faces, but Parkinson's tends to flatten every attempted expression into a grimace of bewilderment. Colin shoots me closer, using an old large-format film camera with vintage black and white stock. I have been starting to feel very iffy today – the tickle at the back of the throat, mild sweats – so I don't imagine any of these shots will be useable. I can feel my head filling up with fluid.

By showtime, I'm feeling decidedly rubbish and afterwards I'm in my bunk early. But I can't sleep – my throat's too sore and the bus keeps stopping and starting. After a while, I realise that we've broken down and throw jeans on to pop downstairs for a look. There's an emergency van behind us in a narrow lay-by, its orange lights flashing over a field of stubble. I go back to bed around 5 a.m. to be woken by Derek at

8.30 to be told that a replacement bus will be arriving shortly. We form a human chain to move the bedding, bags and beers from bus to bus and are on the road again by ten. Not too much of a drama. It would all have been far more stressful in the rain or snow. My cold has shifted further down my windpipe this morning, heading into my lungs. My voice is now much more affected than last night. At least it's only one more show. But the day off in Exeter is gone now. A relief, in a way. I don't think I can take another gallery or museum or cathedral. I intend to see only the inside of a duvet.

DAY 96, Bude, Cornwall, UK

I play some music in my high-ceilinged hotel room in an Exeter I have not set foot in, let alone explored. The music does little to revive. Last night, I ate room service in bed, watched a Cary Grant movie and slumbered deep within the surreal caverns and hallways of my infection. But I'm a little better than yesterday, when my voice had dropped an octave into Lee Marvin territory. Mr Fudge has kindly bought meds from the chemist this morning and I gub a couple of paracetamol. What will be will be.

We arrive at The Wyldes around midday and a kindly young bloke in catering furnishes me with a comforting baked potato and vegan chilli. It's fresh, homemade fare and very welcome after the last few days of not even *finding* the catering zone. The venue is a purpose-built little outdoor place in the backwoods of north Cornwall. The dressing rooms are set around a small courtyard of wooden shacks like a silent film studio lot. Kris lives round these parts and arrives with family in tow an hour later, young Rosie looking well-recovered after her hospitalisation last week with what turned out to be severe tonsilitis. I remember that feeling well, being prone to successive bouts of infection until they whipped out my tonsils and adenoids when I was five. The toxic drip from throat to stomach, the agony of swallowing – I'm grateful the doctors took action. Before the op, they put me and another boy onto trollies and wheeled us to a big side room full of soft toys. The floor was covered in teddy bears and stuffed Disney characters. I took a dim view of this, reasoning quite logically that this overkill of reassurance portended extreme unpleasantness. The anaesthetist had me count up to ten as he applied the terrifying leather face mask. I zonked out at seven and awoke feeling very sore and confused. That's the last time I had a general anaesthetic and I hope it stays that way. And people tell me ketamine is fun. Fuck off.

I take a stroll around the site. It's a flat patch of grassland with a coppice of silver birch at the back. Very dainty. I speak to Sam, the owner/promoter, and get a potted history. His father farmed his whole life, but as his Parkinson's advanced in his eighties, he allowed his kids to develop the land in new directions. He tells me the trees were planted with a forestry grant, but their wood is no use for much other than matchsticks. And they're not birch – but he can't remember what they are. Never let the facts get in the way of the story. Lights are strung from the branches and I make a plan to watch the Minds from here. Sam goes about his business, moving seating around, then marching off with a ladder under his arm. It's a family affair and so far it feels like bliss.

Soundcheck is better than expected. My voice has a weird edge to it and I can't quite manoeuvre it the way I'm used to. The vibrato is not there. I don't even want to think about the top notes. I'll just give it everything and pray it doesn't pack in before the end of tonight's scheduled one-hour set. The Minds crew slouch about in the backstage courtyard, relaxed and cheerful. The warm June sun is beaming down from on high. There's a smaller local stage set up alongside the main platform, and a band with a sax player and a girl singer strike up making an acceptable racket. Everyone's enjoying the weather. We will leave on the bus bound for home at ten-thirty. No chance to say goodbye to Jim, Charlie, Cherisse, Gordy, Ged, Erik and the regal Sarah Brown. They've been a delight to tour alongside. I'm sorry to see this little circus go. On the big bookshelf in our living room growing up, there was a thick paperback of my mum's, written about the Hollywood silent era. *The Parade's Gone By.*

As I walk in the darkness to the bus with my gear from the dressing room, I get talking to a security guard, whose accent I recognise as Leicestershire. He tells me he was in the army but got 'blown up' in Northern Ireland. He proves to be extremely helpful extricating our bus from a tight space in the dark and helping us hook onto our trailer. I am several beers in when it becomes apparent that all is not right with our main driver, who was spotted earlier pissed and talking bollocks. He's now in no condition to assist the inexperienced second driver, who is to drive the first leg of the journey to Glasgow.

I decide to stay up all night drinking which, in the circumstances, proves to be a wise decision. Our first driver is fired by his company and dumped at a train station somewhere in the north of England while the second driver has to drop us at Carlisle, having run out of hours. We drag ourselves to the station and Iain buys us first-class tickets home. I keep drinking beer. I get home and keep drinking beer with Luke. By midnight I am done, and consequently spend most of the next three weeks in bed, coughing like a consumptive. It's the sickest I've ever been. A year ago, we had just started out on that epic American tour. I guess it all finally hit me. Sometimes you need to stop. But every time I stop, I fear I will never start again.

OUTRO

At the end of *The Incredible Shrinking Man*, our hero faces an uncertain future. Having been reduced to the size of an ant, he has just successfully fought off a house spider using a needle as a spear. As the film closes, he contemplates the battles ahead at a cellular scale with what can only be described as a kind of sanguine wonder. Those of us with degenerative conditions have a small element of that insouciant fatalism. We can see that all lives are degenerating – yours along with ours – and that we just have a little more of a clue about the nature and structure of our decline. And there are always worse conditions to have. For example, I wouldn't relish having a death match with a giant arachnid every day for the rest of my life.

Besides, none of us wants to peer too far into the future, as can be witnessed by humankind's three-wise-monkeys approach to climate catastrophe. We cling desperately on to the present, driven by this affliction that no matter how bad it gets, things will turn out alright. Even when we know we're headed inexorably for hell, we find faith in a dream of the opposite. This very stupidity drives me on. The graveyards groan with smart suicides. The rest of us make merry in our wilful disregard of the facts. No matter how far my affliction advances, a last remaining part of me will insist it's all been a mistake. One day, I'll come to, twenty-six again, setting out on this adventure with a band and a bass guitar, fit as fiddle, strong as an ox. Open your eyes, lad – opportunity knocks.

ACKNOWLEDGEMENTS

This book itself has been an essential therapy. Like Edward St Aubin's Patrick Melrose novels, the action of putting one's life onto the page is catharsis enough. If in doubt, write it down. Words, even more than music, are a balm; they expose the central truth of our lives.

Pete Selby, editor and publisher, has for some insane reason not seen fit to excise most of these meanderings, and he and his team's very precise advice (especially that of James Lilford) has been gratefully appreciated. Alex Green, my wonderful novelist friend, has been an irrepressible inspiration. This book would not have existed without the sage and tender guidance of Del Amitri's manager Andy Prevezer.

I do have to thank Phil Smith for the title and I must recognise my mother, Barbara, who encouraged my sisters and I to read. The essential alarm of that wonderful woman is forever a guiding light. My Love, Emma, has been the grounding force of my life, and of course her, and my, son Luke a crucial and wise component of the words written here. Lastly, Iain Harvie, my partner and companion through this seemingly endless journey, has been both brother and colleague, a towering pillar of a man without whom I am merely an idea.

THE END

The team at New Modern would like to thank the following individuals:

Nige Tassell for copy-editing
Peter Stoneman for proofreading and editorial support
Marie Doherty for typesetting
Paul Palmer-Edwards for cover design
Colin Constance for author and cover photos
Andy Prevezer for artist management
Dusty Miller for publicity